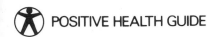 POSITIVE HEALTH GUIDE

 KU-783-377

THE BRITISH SCHOOL OF OSTEOPATHY
1-4 SUFFOLK ST., LONDON SW1Y 4HG
TEL: 01 - 930 9254-8

CONQUERING PAIN

How to overcome the discomfort of arthritis, backache, migraine, heart disease, childbirth, period pain and many other common conditions

Dr Sampson Lipton
MB, ChB, DARCS (Eng), FFARCS (Eng)

MARTIN DUNITZ

To the Pain Relief Foundation, Walton Hospital, Liverpool, England

© Sampson Lipton 1984

First published in the United Kingdom in 1984
by Martin Dunitz Ltd, London

All rights reserved. No part of this publication
may be reproduced, stored in a retrieval system, or transmitted,
in any form or by any means, without the prior permission of the
publisher.

British Library Cataloguing-in-Publication Data

Lipton, Sampson
   Conquering pain. – (Positive health guide)
   1. Pain
   I. Title II. Series
   616.0472   RD81

   ISBN 0–906348–63–3
   ISBN 0–906348–62–5 Pbk

Phototypeset in Garamond by Input Typesetting Ltd, London
Printed and bound in Singapore

Dr Sampson Lipton, MB, ChB, DARCS (Eng), FFARCS (Eng)

At the time of writing, Dr Lipton was Director of the Centre for Pain Relief at Walton Hospital, Liverpool. He recently retired from that position but continues to be Honorary Medical Director of the Pain Relief Foundation. He is also a Committee Member of the International Association for the Study of Pain, and Trustee of the Pain Relief Foundation. In 1980–1 he was Hunterian Professor, Royal College of Surgeons.

He teaches and lectures extensively around the world, especially in Australia, New Zealand and North America. In 1979–80 he helped the Pain Relief Centres at the Royal Brisbane Hospital and at the University of Otago in Dunedin. In 1981 he lectured in various aspects of pain relief at the University of Western Australia, and gave seminars, lectures and demonstrations at the University of Queensland. Dr Lipton worked for most of the latter half of 1983 as Visiting Professor at Texas Tech University's Pain Relief Center in Lubbock.

He has edited and contributed to numerous medical books, and is the author of two, including *The Control of Chronic Pain*. In addition, Dr Lipton has published over thirty specialist papers.

In 1982 Dr Lipton was awarded the prestigious Merseyside Gold Medal for outstanding achievements during the last twenty-five years as Director of the Centre for Pain Relief.

CONTENTS

INTRODUCTION

Pain is the commonest reason by far that makes people seek help from their doctors. But not everybody feels pain; there are a few people who are born with an inability to appreciate the sensation. At first, you might think that it is a good thing not to have to experience the pain of, for example, an injury or a toothache. However, imagine what would happen if that injury were severe enough to break a bone and you did not know it, or the toothache went on to become an abcess and you did not realize it until the swelling of your face became very noticeable.

Being able to feel pain is a great safeguard in our lives. It enables us to have some chance of surviving from childhood to adult life and then to go on living so that we may protect our own children. Pain is, therefore, normally of great benefit. It only becomes a disadvantage if, after giving us warning of an injury, it then goes on and on and does not disappear; it is no longer serving any useful purpose. This is what is called chronic or intractable pain, and it is one of the most difficult symptoms that medical science has had to learn to deal with.

The practice of medicine probably began when one person went to another, saying, 'I've got a pain. Help me.' However, it was not until the 1940s that anything could be done for many illnesses except to make the sufferers as comfortable as possible. Before then, most medical treatment just helped the body's own recuperative powers to deal with an illness. Surgery was available but, compared to today, it was of a simple kind. Great impetus was given to medicine during and after the Second World War when effective anaesthesia and the control of infections with antibiotics were introduced.

Since then, modern medicine has been so effective in dealing with the causes of disease and disability that the control of pain was pushed into the background and only recently has any scientific attention been paid to it. Not only has this meant that sufferers of chronically painful conditions such as backache, arthritis and headache had to put up with their aches and pain as best they could, but that even the pain which occurs after surgical operations was not very well treated. Fortunately, times have changed and new methods and drugs are now available. Best of all, there is a growing realization among the medical profession that a lot still remains to be done in this area of health, and specialized units – such as the Pain Relief Centre in Liverpool of which I am director – are being set up to deal with the difficult problem of chronic pain. We see around 2,500 patients each year at our clinic, and have treated nearly every type of acute and chronic pain. Even so, there are not nearly enough of these units to deal with the number of people suffering from pain.

The effects of pain on people have a great impact on society. For example, about 30 per cent of the British population suffers from headache at some time during any one year. The incidence of backache, too, is quite remarkable: the Arthritis and Rheumatism Council of Great Britain estimate that about 20 million working days are lost each year because of it. Pain is responsible for a huge expenditure on painkilling drugs and for loss of income due to absence from work. In the United States, some $2 billion are spent on these drugs each year while, until quite recently, less than $1 million was spent on research into alleviating pain.

The same proportion holds true in Britain and other Western countries, and the Third World is even worse off with little prospect of change in the near future.

There is a great deal that you can do to avoid and alleviate your own pain and that of others, and I shall be discussing this later. First, however, I want to describe what pain actually is, what causes it and how it travels from its point of origin to the brain, where you feel it.

1. WHAT IS PAIN?

It is not very easy to say exactly what is meant by 'pain' because there are so many different types. Just think of back pain, the pain of a broken bone and of a heart attack, or that caused by a scald or by migraine, and it is easy to see that each pain has its own characteristics. One type may be constant, another comes in waves, one occurs in agonizing bursts, one feels like an iron band around the chest or head, and so on. Each is different yet well recognized when it recurs.

What causes pain?

According to the International Association for the Study of Pain, 'Pain is a warning sign to the body that some part of it is being damaged.' There are a variety of ways in which damage or potential damage can be done to body tissues. It can happen when a part of the body is cut, torn or crushed. It can be caused by heat or cold, or it can be due to chemicals. The chemicals may be thrown on the skin surface and damage it as might happen with an acid, or the chemicals may be produced by the body itself as in arthritis or migraine.

Pain receptors Once the body is damaged, pain is transmitted from the skin or another part of the body by small electric currents along nerves. In your body, you have many special sense organs called receptors which are mainly concentrated in the skin, although they are situated in most other parts. These receptors are sensi-

tive to changes in your body; they send messages to the brain to inform it if it is hot or cold, if your skin, say, is pressing upon something, and pass on other information besides. There is a difference, though, between a painless pressure on the skin and pressure that damages it by crushing. The first is useful information, but the other is urgent information, telling the brain to move that part of the skin from the thing that is crushing it as soon as possible.

In general, the receptors which activate the electrical messages to the brain are of two basic types: those which send general information (called 'non-noxious information' by scientists) and those which send information about damage ('noxious information'). An organ which sends electrical messages concerning damage or injury is known as a pain receptor, or nociceptor.

These pain receptors are subdivided into mechanoreceptors (those which inform the brain about crushing and tearing), thermoreceptors (which deal with heat and cold) and non-specific receptors (which detect a variety of sensations), and between them they respond to all forms of pain. In addition, other types of receptors are involved in sending information about sensations we might feel, so that the body can tell the difference between, say, a burn produced by a red-hot, sharp needle and that made by a cigarette. It is merely that different receptors are involved in the electrical signals.

Although the majority of pain receptors are located in your skin, there are also receptors inside your body. The type of pain you may feel there depends on the types of receptors that are present and the signals they send. Take the intestines, for example: they have almost no receptors to detect crushing, tearing or burning, so that the intestines can be cut, crushed or burned without our feeling it very much. However, if they are distended with gas (wind) or if they contract violently, they are very painful indeed. Because of this lack of receptors, pain that occurs deep in your body is difficult to point to exactly – in other words, it is not well localized – but you can usually tell whether it is in the centre of the abdomen or to one side. You can also feel when you get spasm (a sudden, painful contraction of the muscles) of the gut – the 'gripes' as it is often called.

Your muscles respond to different pain receptors, especially those which detect waste chemicals produced in the body by exercise. Normally these are washed away by the bloodstream, but in some people the circulation has been damaged by disease and these waste products remain in the muscle. They are detected by receptors and the brain registers pain. This happens in heart disease when the lack of blood to the heart muscle leaves waste products that cause pain in these muscles, called angina (see page 57).

Chemicals produced in your body Your body produces a number of other chemicals which cause pain, but they all act by stimulating pain receptors. A good example are those which cause the pain of rheumatic diseases such as arthritis, or inflammation of the joints. Wherever there is inflammation, certain chemicals called kinins are naturally produced by the body, and these stimulate the pain receptors in that area.

However, this is not the whole story since inflammation also stimulates the formation of another substance in the tissues: prostaglandin. This is produced in all sorts of tissues and acts on cells very close to where it is produced, usually working within seconds and then disappearing. There are many types of prostaglandin and not all or even most of them are concerned with pain. In the case of the one produced by inflammation, it triggers three things: the blood vessels widen, causing redness; these vessels leak fluid, causing swelling; and the pain receptors become even more sensitive so that the nerve impulses are created more easily and thus pain is increased.

Not only that, but the rate of production of the prostaglandin is itself increased by the presence of kinins. This type of action often occurs in the body and is known as 'positive feedback' – one substance produces a second and then the second affects the first. It is a vicious circle and this is one of the explanations for why the pain in inflammation gets worse and worse. Fortunately, there are drugs such as aspirin which are antiprostaglandins. They prevent the formation of prostaglandin so that, gradually, the whole painful process winds down. That is why aspirin is such a useful anti-inflammatory drug (see Chapter 10).

Another type of prostaglandin is produced in women which causes the muscles of the uterus to contract. This is vital in childbirth, but an imbalance of this chemical may also cause a woman to develop pains during menstruation. This period pain – dysmenorrhoea – is discussed in Chapter 8.

How your body 'feels' pain
The sensation of pain is perceived in your brain, but before this happens, the electrical impulses produced by the receptors in your body must travel along nerve fibres to the spinal cord and then to the brain.

There are three different types of nerve fibres that detect pain and other sensations. Only pain is carried by the numerous thin C fibres which form a network under the skin; while the fewer and thicker A-beta (Aβ) fibres carry most of the other sensations, such as touch, pressure and position. There are also the relatively thin A-delta (Aδ) fibres, some of which can carry pain, and they act in much the same way as the C fibres. However, C fibres are able to regrow if they are damaged. For example, if an area of skin is destroyed by a burn, both types of fibres are also destroyed; but when the skin heals, C fibres from the surrounding undamaged skin will eventually grow back into the previously burned area and re-form the C-fibre network. The A fibres do not have this ability, and they also tend to decrease in number as you grow older. This makes diseases which destroy A fibres, such as shingles (see pages 89–90), more painful in old age than they are when you are younger. The reason why is tied up with the relationship between the A-beta and the C fibres, which is also important for pain relief. When the skin is damaged, signals are sent along all the nerves, especially the C and A-beta fibres. At the spine, where all these signals come together, the non-painful signals from the A-beta fibres tend to block the painful ones travelling along the C fibres. This is known as 'gate control', and is one way your body is able to cut down pain. Several methods of pain relief are based on gate control, and I shall be describing these in Chapters 11 and 12.

Interaction between pain-carrying C nerve fibres and the faster-acting A-beta fibres results in less pain stimulation reaching the brain.

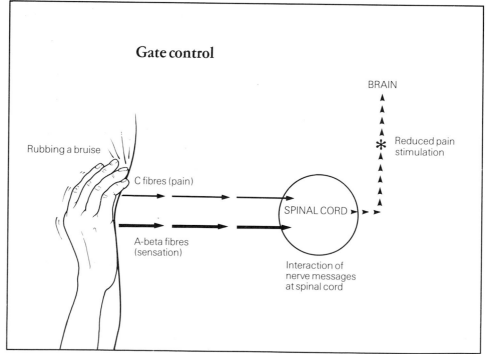

Gate control

BRAIN

Reduced pain stimulation

Rubbing a bruise

C fibres (pain)

SPINAL CORD

A-beta fibres (sensation)

Interaction of nerve messages at spinal cord

First and second pains The existence of these different types of nerve fibres is responsible for the different types of pain you feel. If you prick your foot with a needle, for example, you will almost immediately feel a sharp pain. Then, after a short interval, you will usually feel an aching, dull pain which spreads over an area larger than the part of the foot you pricked with the needle. In addition, this ache does not disappear quickly like the sharp pain, but only gradually fades away. These two types of pain are called 'first pains' and 'second pains', and they are the results of the activities of the different types of nerve fibres. (Some people, though, do not ever feel the second pain and this is not abnormal.)

When part of the body is damaged – as with the pinprick – all the nerve endings in that area are activated and send signals to the brain. The A fibres act very quickly – almost instantaneously – taking the 'first' pain (in this case, the sharp prick of the needle) to be recognized by the brain, and shortly afterwards, the C fibres relay their message – the 'second' pain (the dull ache) – to the brain. The table below compares the speeds at which the messages are transmitted along the fibres.
The different types of fibres interact with each other, and, as we have seen, the A fibres can modify the pain we feel by partially blocking the C fibres.

What happened to one of my patients clearly illustrates the way in which first and second pains occur. It was winter with snow and some ice on the ground, and Bert stepped outside one morning to clear a path to his car parked in the road. He did not take quite as much care as he should have,

his feet slipped out from under him and down he went. Naturally, he stuck out an arm to save himself, and he broke his wrist when his full weight came down on it. This type of broken wrist is very common and is called a Colles' fracture, after the nineteenth-century surgeon who first described it.

During the last icy spell, we treated no less than twenty-seven Colles' fractures at my hospital, and some of these even happened to patients coming to or going from the hospital! Like Bert, all these people felt the same things at the same time as, and immediately after, sustaining the fractures. First, they felt a sharp pain as the bone broke. Some of the patients could describe how the whole incident happened as if in slow motion. They felt the increasing pressure put on their wrists as their hands and arms took the weight of their bodies, culminating in a tremendously sharp pain as the break occurred. This first pain lasted for perhaps as long as one minute and then the second pain began. This was much duller and spread over the whole fracture site and into the lower part of the forearm and into the hand. Over a period of fifteen minutes or more, the pain became increasingly intense, and stayed at this level except when it became a sharp pain during movement of the fracture. This additional pain was the first pain again, due to movement of the broken bone. Most pains follow this pattern.

The reflexes In addition to the work of the A fibres in quickly identifying pain – and therefore potential or actual damage to the body – there is another system which allows you to take action as fast as possible to remove any part

• **A-beta (Aβ) fibres**	90–100 m/sec =	180–200 miles (290–320 km) per hour
• **A-delta (Aδ) fibres**	20 m/sec =	40 miles (64 km) per hour
• **C fibres**	less than 1 m/sec =	2¼ miles (3.6 km) per hour

of your body from damage. This is called 'reflex action'. A reflex has three basic parts: the receptor that receives the warning; the nerve pathway to and from the spinal cord; and the effector, which is a part of the body that responds to the warning. Together these three parts form what is known as the 'reflex arc'.

Your reflexes react so quickly because the electrical impulse produced by the receptor travels over a very short nerve pathway – only as far as the spinal cord – so your conscious thought does not enter into the movement. A good example of a reflex action is when you put your hand on a hot pan and immediately snatch it away before you consciously realize that the pan is hot. In other words, the thought of what you did only strikes you after you did it. This type of reflex consists of a signal from the burned fingers that something unpleasant and dangerous is happening. This signal is sent along a nerve to the spinal cord which immediately sends back signals to muscles in the arm which snatch the hand away from the danger. While this action is going on, other signals make their way, more slowly, up to the brain. Only when they reach it do you understand what has happened and feel pain.

How long will the pain last? Normally after removing the cause of the pain, it settles down after a longer or shorter time. In the case of burns (and many other injuries) the pain will only completely disappear when healing is well advanced. The time-scale for a pain tends to depend on the cause of the pain and the effect that it has on the tissues of the body.

To continue with the previous example, a small burn involving the end of a finger will not produce as much pain, nor will it last as long, as the pain produced from a burn involving the whole hand. Thus you can expect to take longer to heal and to suffer more with the large burn than with the smaller one.

Referred pain In addition to the different types of pain, you might also experience pain in a part of your body even though the cause for it is in a completely different place. This is called 'referred pain', and it comes about because of the way the central nervous system is constructed and because of the way the nerves are distributed around the body.

Damage is commonly done to the inner side of the elbow – the 'funny bone' – either through a blow or by leaning on the elbow too much. In either case, the pain is felt in the little finger, and not in the elbow at all. This is because the brain, which picks up the impulse from the pain receptor in the elbow, does not recognize that particular point on the nerve in the elbow, but only that some sort of damage has been done to that particular pathway. In this case, the brain always interprets that pain as coming from the little finger.

The reason why some pains are referred can be traced back to the way you developed in the womb. In the foetus, many of the organs first start growing in places from which they will travel to another part of the body. For instance, the diaphragm – the muscular wall which divides the abdomen from the heart and lungs – begins life in the region that will become the shoulder. After it descends to its permanent position, it leaves behind its original nerves, and in later life, if damage is done to the diaphragm, the pain will be felt in the shoulder. Since the membrane surrounding the lungs and heart is connected to the diaphragm, any pain arising from either – pleurisy in the lower lung or a coronary thrombosis (heart attack), for instance – tends to be felt in the shoulder area.

As well as the way in which the nervous system is constructed, the way in which the nerves are placed throughout the body will also result in referred pain. Pain from a slipped disc may be felt down the leg or in the arm because the nerves to these areas arise in that part of the spinal cord which is under pressure (see page 46). Also, if the muscles within 2–3 in (5–7.5 cm) of the spine are damaged, the pain will be felt near the centre of the spine, but damaged muscles a little further away will refer pain to the side of the body.

There is a great deal more to pain than just its physical origins. Psychological factors, such as your mood and personality, greatly affect the way you experience pain. It is these that I want to examine in the next chapter.

A knock on a sensory nerve refers pain and tingling to the spot from where the nerve is coming – in this example, from the little finger.

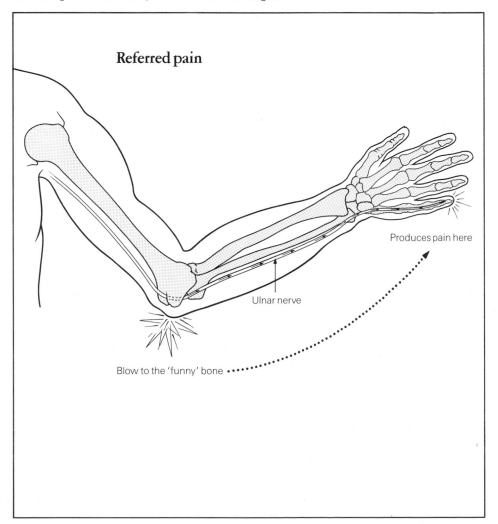

Referred pain

Produces pain here

Ulnar nerve

Blow to the 'funny' bone

2. PAIN AND THE MIND

Pain tolerance and pain thresholds

People do not experience pain in the same way. There is a variation in all our senses so that some people appreciate them a great deal and others only with difficulty. For example, some are born with very keen eyesight and can see things quite clearly at remarkable distances, while the vast majority of us cannot. In the same way, some people feel pain easily and others do not. This is called 'pain tolerance', and is why some people are able to stand more pain than others. Your pain tolerance can affect your behaviour, as the following example shows.

Two cars collide on a slippery street. Both drivers have been shaken up – both physically and mentally – about the same amount, but one continues on his way to work, while the other feels so much pain that he hails a taxi and goes straight to his doctor. The second driver is not exaggerating his pain – he really does feel it – but he unfortunately has a much lower pain tolerance than the first driver.

There is nothing that can be done to change this type of variation between two human beings. But this is a rather extreme example, as relatively few people are completely oblivious to pain – or completely prostrated by it. Most of us feel it to the same degree and can bear about the same amount.

Your pain threshold is a different matter. It is the point at which you first feel pain, and this is pretty equal in everyone. For instance, if you gradu-ally push an object, say a pencil, on to the skin, you will tend to feel the first discomfort (the pain threshold) at much the same pressure as everyone else would. To continue the example, keep pressing the pencil down and steadily increase the pressure. Each person will reach a different stage when they want it taken away – in other words, they have reached their pain tolerance level.

Although pain thresholds tend to be the same in most cultures, the levels of pain tolerance can vary radically. The extraordinary amounts of pain that can be borne by some groups is well known: during the sacred Sun Dance, the North American Plains Indians have skewers inserted into their chests which are then pulled upon. In East Africa, people have parts of their scalps removed without anaesthetic so that the underlying skulls can be examined by a *doktari*. However, to a far less degree, more common cultural attributes such as the traditional English 'stiff upper lip' and the emotional reactions of certain Mediterranean groups will have a great effect on these people's ability to tolerate pain. These are examples of learned behaviour, or social conditioning, and we are subjected to this from earliest childhood.

In addition, what you learn as an individual in your first years will also have a significant impact on the way you react to things that cause pain. Children whose parents react with excessive shows of sympathy every time their offspring suffers the slightest knock or discomfort, gradually learn by repeated experience that having a pain, however minor, invariably brings love and sympathy. These children tend to become adults who are inclined to let those around them know in intimate detail about every ache and pain they experience. It is not that their pain tolerance level is lower than that of someone who generally keeps a 'stiff upper lip', it is simply that they have learnt to react to their pain differently.

How pain can be 'blocked out'

Sometimes you may not notice a pain, when on another occasion that pain, caused by the same thing, bothers you a great deal. I have already mentioned in the previous chapter one way that the body physically modifies pain – by controlling painful sensation along the thin C nerve fibres by blocking some of it with the larger A nerve fibres. This is only one example of what is called 'modulation' in our nervous systems. There are many ways of modulating the different types of impulses your nerves transmit, and these modulations are designed either to be life-protecting or to cut out unwanted information. Often they have a psychological basis.

One example is when a person escapes from a burning room and only afterwards feels pain from the burns received while getting out. Because the most important thing was to save his life, the sensation of pain was completely suppressed until later. Sometimes this type of suppression occurs when you concentrate very hard. Painful sensations may not reach your consciousness at all and there is no room for them until your concentration is broken. The ball player who catches the ball and then scores may not realize that he has broken a finger until much later on, when the pain is so bad that he cannot even pick up a pencil, much

less a ball. A more serious example is that which was first noticed during the Second World War. Soldiers on the battlefield often did not notice the pain of very serious wounds until relatively long after they were removed from the action. Some did not even feel the pain of amputation. The exact reason for this is unclear, but certainly their concentration on survival seemed to have blocked out the pain.

Another way in which your sensations are automatically controlled is due to the way your nervous system is arranged. You are continually receiving a vast amount of information sent to your nervous system – your brain and spinal cord – from your skin, muscles, eyes, ears and so on. And if all this information were allowed to go straight into your conscious brain, you would be completely overwhelmed by it. Since much of this information is not important, there is no point in a great deal of it reaching conscious level and, in fact, most of it does not. There is no reason for you consciously to know that, when you are excited, your blood pressure is rising, as that can be taken care of automatically without your actually realizing it. On the other hand, although you do not normally bother about the temperature of your skin, if you sit in a cold draught, you soon realize what has happened. Because your brain knows that this situation is not a good one for your body, the sensation of a cold skin is allowed to rise into your consciousness and you do something about it – you move.

This process of modulation goes on continually, with most of the information that reaches your nervous system never reaching your mind. Because your body varies the amount of information that is sent to your conscious brain, modulation alters from time to time. What is allowed to rise into your mind depends on what you are doing at the time, how much you are concentrating on something else and how important this information is to you.

If you have severe chronic pain, you can learn to use this modulation to your advantage. By immersing yourself in work, exciting games, books and films or by just watching an interesting programme on television, you can distract your conscious mind from recognizing pain. One famous actress was able to make the pain of arthritis vanish while absorbed in performing her role on stage, and dentists have found that their patients bear the pain of drilling much better if they are listening to music they enjoy.

Measuring pain

Although pain is basically a subjective experience, it can be measured, but with some difficulty and within limits. The simplest method is to use what is termed a Visual Analogue Scale or VAS for short (see illustration opposite). We often use the VAS at the Pain Relief Centre in Liverpool. This involves giving the person whose pain you want to measure a piece of paper with a line drawn on it, and asking him to imagine that the line represents his pain. At one end of the line, there is no pain at all, while the other end represents the worst possible pain that the person can ever imagine. In other words, the line is a personal or subjective thermometer of pain.

The person is asked to make a mark on the line at a point which he thinks measures the amount of pain he has at that particular time. The VAS line is usually standardized at 4 in (10 cm) long; the length of the line which represents the person's pain can then be measured with a ruler, and by comparing the measurements made on different days, it is a very easy way of recording that person's pain from day to day. The only problem with this method – and it is a problem that is

present with almost all measurements of pain – is that it is only reliable for one person at a time. It is of no use in comparing one person's pain against another's. The reason for this is that, as we have already seen, people differ in their appreciation of pain. Nevertheless, the VAS is a very good method if you want to keep a record of your own pain. Sometimes it is useful to do this to see if a new treatment or drug is helping.

Another simple method of recording your pain is merely to make a note at the same time each day as to whether the pain is the same, worse or better than the day before. A variation of this is to give numbers to the amount of pain – 0 to 10 is the usual range – and this is really a VAS without the line. The scale can be shortened to 0, 1, 2 and 3, with 0 meaning no pain and 3 meaning very severe pain, with 1 and 2 somewhere in between. Often this method or a variation of it is used by patients attending pain relief clinics like ours, so that some idea of the variation of the pain, its strength and how long it lasts can be obtained by the specialist.

The McGill Pain Questionnaire

It is possible to get a more accurate idea of the level of pain, and to compare this with others'. Sometimes I want to find out the type and strength of pain that a person may be suffering, and in that case I give the patient a list of groups of words, each group representing a particular type of pain. For instance, the words of one group may be 'flickering, quivering, pulsing, throbbing, beating, pounding', and the person is asked to pick the one that best describes his pain. This is known as the McGill Pain Questionnaire (see illustration on page 18), and it was devised by Ronald Melzack, a professor of psychology at McGill University in Canada.

There are twenty groups of words,

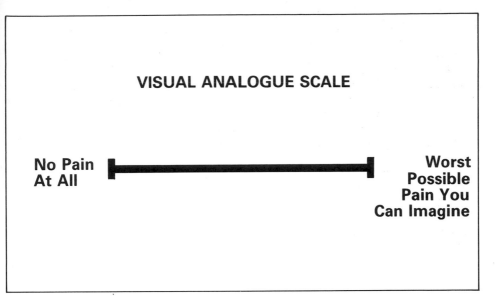

VISUAL ANALOGUE SCALE

No Pain At All ———————————————— Worst Possible Pain You Can Imagine

The visual analogue scale (VAS) provides a simple way of measuring pain. You make a mark on the line according to how bad your pain feels.

and if the words in one or more groups do not fit the pain, the patient does not select any in that group or groups. The words are graded in intensity, and when totalling the final score, the positions of the words selected are added together – so many firsts, seconds, thirds and so on within a group – the lower down within a group, the higher the score. Thus an overall pain intensity can be calculated, which, to some extent, can be compared from person to person.

This questionnaire is divided into different sections because different people have different reactions to pain. Some are not worried by it, for example, while others are very nervous. Groups 1 to 10 are the sensory words – what the patient actually feels. Groups 11 to 15 assess the effect of the pain on the person – what they think about it – while Group 16 is similar to this but in a broader sense. Groups 17 to 20 comprise the miscellaneous descriptions which do not fit elsewhere.

These words were originally selected by asking patients in pain to describe what they felt. It was then noticed that different people tended to use the same words to describe their pain, and that even people in different countries tended to use the same words or very close equivalents. Furthermore, when the various people interviewed were asked to put these words in order of discomfort or intensity, they all tended to place them in a very similar order.

There is one added feature in the McGill Pain Questionnaire. You will see a section at the bottom of the list, labelled 'PPI', which is the abbreviation for 'present pain intensity'. The patients are asked to fill in their estimate of the level of their pain at that moment, on a simple scale of 0 to 5. This is similar to the previously mentioned do-it-yourself methods.

Because the McGill questionnaire gives a measure of the overall intensity of a particular type of pain as well as information about what a pain feels like, it is possible to compare the relative severity of different types of pain suffered by people who have completed the questionnaire. You can see the re-

McGILL-MELZACK PAIN QUESTIONNAIRE

1
Flickering
Quivering
Pulsing
Throbbing
Beating
Pounding

2
Jumping
Flashing
Shooting

3
Pricking
Boring
Drilling
Stabbing
Lancinating

4
Sharp
Cutting
Lacerating

5
Pinching
Pressing
Gnawing
Cramping
Crushing

6
Tugging
Pulling
Wrenching

7
Hot
Burning
Scalding
Searing

8
Tingling
Itchy
Smarting
Stinging

9
Dull
Sore
Hurting
Aching
Heavy

10
Tender
Taut
Rasping
Splitting

11
Tiring
Exhausting

12
Sickening
Suffocating

13
Fearful
Frightful
Terrifying

14
Punishing
Gruelling
Cruel
Vicious
Killing

15
Wretched
Binding

16
Annoying
Troublesome
Miserable
Intense
Unbearable

17
Spreading
Radiating
Penetrating
Piercing

18
Tight
Numb
Drawing
Squeezing
Tearing

19
Cool
Cold
Freezing

20
Nagging
Nauseating
Agonizing
Dreadful
Torturing

PPI
0 No pain
1 Mild
2 Discomforting
3 Distressing
4 Horrible
5 Excruciating

Constant
Periodic
Brief

This questionnaire enables researchers to compare to some extent people's levels of pain. Each descriptive word carries its own score – the lower down in its group, the higher its value. The sum of the scores gives what is termed a person's 'pain rating index' – in other words, their overall pain intensity. The final 'present pain intensity' (PPI) section gives an idea of the pain level at the moment the questionnaire is completed.

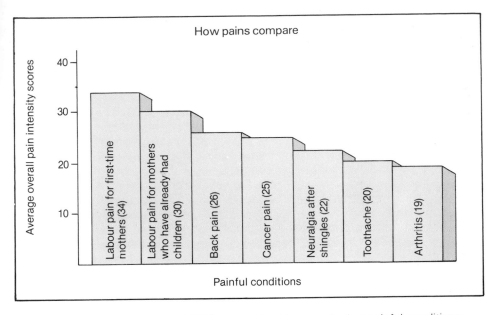

Average overall pain intensity scores

40 —

30 —

20 —

10 —

Labour pain for first-time mothers (34)

Labour pain for mothers who have already had children (30)

Back pain (26)

Cancer pain (25)

Neuralgia after shingles (22)

Toothache (20)

Arthritis (19)

Painful conditions

Average total 'pain rating index' (PRI) scores for labour and other painful conditions. These were obtained by Prof Melzack and others using the McGill Questionnaire.

sults of Prof Melzack and others' 1981 research in the graph above, which shows that labour pains in women having their first or subsequent babies – are among the most intense pains suffered by people who have completed the questionnaire.

I shall be covering some of the different conditions that cause pain, including childbirth, in later chapters, but it is important to mention here that although the pain of labour ranks high, it is usually more easily coped with than, say, cancer pain, because the woman in labour knows that the pains will last for a limited amount of time and that they are part and parcel of giving birth and that they are not caused by a long-lasting, life-threatening disease.

How mood affects pain

Depression I expect that when you are feeling 'off colour', everyday worries tend to disturb you much more than normal. In exactly the same way, you feel aches and pain much more when you are not at your best. In fact, if you are depressed, you may find that pain and your mood are totally interlinked.

As we have seen, quantifying pain is very difficult because we are trying to measure an experience. Explaining pain becomes even more difficult when someone who apparently has no physical element to their pain, is clearly suffering pain: the pain is all psychological. Patients with neuroses or mental illness are of this type but their pain is no less real to them, and they will show many or all of the responses to pain which appear when a pain of physical origin is present. Even when you are just mildly depressed, you too may find that you develop aches or pains which were not there before.

It is quite well known that people who are in chronic pain become depressed. Pain and depression often go together the other way, too, so that somebody who develops a depressive illness also develops pain. There are some drugs such as the antidepressants which can lift the moods of many patients and these are valuable in treating both depression and pain (see Chapter 10). It is not absolutely clear why there is a connection between these two conditions. However, the drugs which often help to relieve pain are the same drugs which may improve depression. It may be that the pathways of chronic pain and depression – located in the lower part of the brain (called the brain stem) which links the higher centres of the brain with the spinal cord – may overlap to some extent and thus respond to the same type of drugs.

Anxiety Another type of mood which can affect your perception of pain is anxiety – an excessive uneasiness. As with depression, when you are in a state of anxiety you may start to feel pain which has no physiological cause. It is not surprising that you may become even more anxious if you do not know what is causing your pain, if your treatment is not effective, and if you do not know what more can be done. The group of drugs known as the benzodiazepines – of which diazepam (Valium) and chlordiazepoxide (Librium) are the most common – are useful for this type of trouble (see Chapter 10), but the prescribing of these is for your doctor to decide. Self-help and professional treatments for anxiety and depression are explained in full in a companion volume – *Anxiety and Depression* by Prof Robert Priest.

Agitation If you do not know why you have a constant pain and your doctor cannot give a good explanation for it – as he or she often cannot – your anxiety may become somewhat uncontrolled and you may become agitated

and very jittery. When this happens your doctor may well give you some drugs to help you. There are many types of these and they are usually very effective. A common group which is often used is the phenothiazines which act directly on the brain. Again, these can only be prescribed by your doctor, who alone has full knowledge of your condition.

The placebo effect
In the late 1950s, Prof Beecher and others discovered in Boston in the United States that when patients with severe pain were unknowingly given a substance with no painkilling properties (usually a sugar pill or a saline solution) – a placebo – instead of the narcotic painkiller morphine, about 35 per cent of them reported marked relief of pain. This was an especially surprising result, since morphine itself relieved severe pain in only 75 per cent of patients. In more recent studies, it has been found that placebos seem to have half the pain-relieving strength of the real drugs and that they are far more effective in those with severe pain than in those with a more mild variety.

These patients were not imagining their pain. However, it seems that when they were given a placebo, the suggestion that it would help them was also given via the attitudes of the medical staff around them (who also did not know if they were administering a drug or a placebo). Suggestion can have a powerful effect and can do much to instil a more positive attitude in someone who is suffering from chronic pain. That is why optimistic encouragement is so important to sufferers, and why hypnosis can sometimes achieve remarkable results (see Chapter 11). In addition, the giving of any drug or placebo also seems to reduce the anxiety and depression a patient may feel and, as we have seen, these can affect that person's perception of pain. This elimination of anxiety may be responsible for the dramatic reduction in the pain of headaches felt by patients given placebos in a study in 1954 – 52 per cent were helped compared to 35 per cent of those suffering other types of pain.

How acute and chronic pain can affect you

As I mentioned in the introduction to this book, acute pain is a beneficial aspect of human life in that it warns of danger to your body. However, when that pain lasts longer than needed as a warning – in other words, it has become long-term or chronic – it can be very difficult for the person to bear and for a doctor to treat.

In the same way that you feel two different kinds of pain when you prick your finger, for example, you can also suffer from either acute or chronic pain. The difference between the two is simply that a chronic pain lasts longer than an acute one. But the way most people react to an acute pain is very different to the way they will deal with a chronic condition.

When your hand has been hit by a hammer, your immediate reaction is to hold and rub the affected place on your hand. At the same time, your pulse rate rises, you begin to sweat, you become light-headed, your blood pressure falls and you feel faint, your skin becomes pale and many other effects occur. After a while, when your system returns to normal, you are left with a large and painful bruise. Your hand has been X-rayed and nothing has been found to be broken; you are reassured, your hand is bandaged and kept immobile for a few days, and you may not be able to carry out your normal work. But you know it is a temporary matter and you are not worried.

Now suppose that you have a chronic pain, such as painful arthritis in the fingers of both hands. It is obvious that there are differences to the pain of hitting your finger with a hammer, but these are differences of degree only. This time the absence from work is an unknown quantity. When can you return? Will you return? Will they keep your job available for you? You are anxious most of the time, your pressure is low, you sweat a lot, your skin is pale, your pulse fast. Will this pain ever stop? Can the doctor help you? Is he any good? He said that he would fix it last time and that didn't work out – and so on.

Although a chronic pain is often far less intense than an acute one, it is the prospect of the pain continuing for the foreseeable future which gives it its own special severity. This can lead to anxiety, depression and despair – a vicious circle that is difficult to break. However, during the last fifteen years or so, several methods have been discovered that go some way towards interrupting the cycle of chronic pain and give hope of being able to manage such pain better ourselves and to help others to do so. Let's look at these now.

Unlearning pain

Operant conditioning Ever since Pavlov trained his dogs to salivate when a bell rang, indicating that they were soon to get some food, scientists have recognized that people's behaviour can be altered by rewards. When a person has pain, the normal reaction of others is to 'reward' that person in a number of ways. People who normally would not give them the time of day now ask them how they are. They get little gifts; other people do their shopping and, best of all, they do not have to go out to work or do the housework because they are ill and in pain.

It is not surprising that some of these people soon discover that, if they stay in pain, they become 'special' and they avoid much unpleasant hard work. They may – usually quite unconsciously – become 'the painful patient', and they do not get better because their 'well' life is much worse than their 'sick' one.

To some extent, the same thing applies to a patient who is in obvious pain – say, with a chronic backache. He may find that if he grimaces and pulls a face, somebody will give him sympathy and ask if he wants a painkiller. A hand held to the head and a strained expression will get the radio turned off. 'Don't do that – it'll give me a headache', or, 'It'll make my headache even worse' are expressions we have all heard, usually from an invalid, often an elderly parent. But most of us are tempted to 'use' our pain in this way when we are ill and/or in pain.

Anything which affects human behaviour is called by specialists an 'operant'. If an operant produces a good result – a 'reward' – it tends to be repeated. If you groan and have a pained expression, it is likely that somebody will produce a pill, sympathy, company and so on. If you would not normally get these things or at least not get them as quickly, more than likely you will repeat the ploy. It is simply human nature.

In the mid-1960s, W. E. Fordyce, a psychologist in Seattle, Washington, reasoned that what an operant had done, another operant properly applied could undo and so the technique of operant conditioning was born. Patients are checked to make sure that the diagnosis of their chronic pain is correct, and then they go to stay at a special unit. There, their daily intake of painkilling drugs (analgesics) is assessed, divided into doses and then given regularly on a timed basis. In this way everyone on the ward (including the patients) knows that they are getting enough analgesics. These drugs are given in very sweet or bitter fluids so that the patients do not taste the analgesic. They are told that at some stage during their treatment, the dose will be reduced without them being told and they have to agree to this before being accepted on to the programme.

The basic technique is simply the reverse of what happens normally. If patients stay in bed, groan, look in pain and so on – nobody takes any notice of them. Only when they get up, move about, take part in ward activity and are helpful to others, do staff and other patients talk to them and accept them into the 'ward community'. This is operant conditioning designed to get the patient active. It is so alien to doctors and nurses that they have to be specially trained to behave in this way.

At the same time, the patients' drugs are being reduced and then cut completely. This is possible because of the method of giving the drugs in solution and at regular times – they are no longer given as a 'reward' for the patients' pain. Eventually the patients become more active and take few if any drugs, although they are still in pain. They have learned to cope with their pain. Although it might appear a heartless method, it usually doesn't take patients long to get used to the new routine, and in the vast majority of people it achieves very positive results.

Our activity programme The type of programme I have just described takes a considerable amount of time (several months) and a lot of staff. In our pain unit, we do not have the resources to carry out a full operant conditioning programme; instead, we use what we call an activity programme.

The patients come to the special unit for eight hours a day, five days a week. Their drugs are dealt with as previously described, and each day is devoted to getting patients who for years have not been very active back to a more normal and certainly more active routine. In one day, for instance, they will take part in one hour of group physiotherapy, one hour of occupational therapy, one hour of group counselling, one hour of hypnotherapy, one hour of pain relief treatment (see Chapters 11 and 12). They also attend lectures about painful conditions. Possibly the most important sessions are those in which the patients comment on themselves and, most significantly, on each other. After all, if they are 'painful patients' – and at least some of them are – they know all the 'tricks' of getting others to do things. They cannot be fooled, and they can be deadly critics.

This programme continues for one month and there are refreshers at intervals to see how the 'veterans' are getting on. This technique also needs plenty of resources but not as many as a full operant conditioning programme, and we have found it to be very effective in helping people to overcome their pain.

What you can do

As I have already mentioned, the way you experience pain is to a large extent learned behaviour, and dealing with chronic pain involves unlearning this behaviour. Ignoring pain by distracting yourself has already been discussed, and operant conditioning, although basically something which should be carried out by professionals caring for those with chronic pain, can to some extent be applied by the person in pain. The realization of how your behaviour may be affecting how much you are feeling pain can go a long way towards making you more able to deal with it.

If you find that you are staying at home or in bed most of the time and that this gives you all the time in the world to dwell on your pain, you could try to devise a system of rewards – going to see a friend or relative, going to see a good film or going out to a favourite restaurant – so that you will become more active *and* learn to distract your mind from the pain. If you make your pain worse by holding your body in a tense and awkward way, simple methods of relaxation (see Chapter 12) can bring relief.

Trying to develop a more positive attitude can help a great deal. If you and those around you think that you will get better and that you yourself can do something to make this happen, it can be surprising how much better you will be able to bear your pain. Try not to have everything done for you – take an active part in your own treatment.

Some people have found that getting involved in fund-raising for research into their own particular illnesses has enabled them to carry on when, before, they felt that their condition was hopeless. One shining example of this is one of my own patients. Mike, a thirty-nine-year-old computer operator, was paralysed from the waist down after a car crash when he was twenty-five and he still suffers severe pain. After his accident, he turned to yachting and to raising money for a research institute at our Pain Relief Foundation in Liverpool. After sailing around the coast of Britain, at the time of writing he has just completed a sponsored 2,500-mile (4,000-km) solo voyage from south-west England to the Azores and back. While not everybody can do what Mike is attempting, anything that keeps you active, relieves your depression and holds your interest and concentration, will be enormously valuable in helping you cope with your pain.

So far we have looked at pain in general terms. In the next seven chapters I want to consider several common, specific painful conditions, and give suggestions on how you can deal with them. If you decide to skip to the chapter that covers your own particular condition, don't forget that the final three chapters (10–12) include practical information on pain relief that should be of value whatever is causing your pain.

3. ARTHRITIS AND RHEUMATISM

Most people use the terms 'arthritis' and 'rheumatism' almost interchangeably. 'Arthritis', though, refers to an inflammation of a joint (although in some varieties inflammation is not present and sometimes the term 'arthrosis' is used), and 'rheumatism' is a much less precise term, generally referring to aches and pain in muscles, ligaments and tendons. Thus, the term 'soft-tissue rheumatism' is becoming more acceptable in the medical world.

All types of arthritis and soft-tissue rheumatism are grouped as the 'rheumatic diseases', and almost everyone is affected by at least one of these at some stage in their lives. In fact, approximately 8 million people in Britain – around one adult in five – suffer from arthritis. And the numbers are growing, as the population of elderly people increases year by year. The pain of arthritis generally tends to be aching and gnawing most of the time rather than sharp and stabbing (see diagram opposite above), and is ranked lower in intensity than the pain of some other conditions such as backache and toothache, according to recent research in Canada (see also diagram on page 19). But as every sufferer knows, the long-term nature of arthritis can make the pain especially hard to live with. Fortunately, there is much that your doctor and you can do to help alleviate the pain, and I shall be describing professional treatment and self-help measures at the end of this chapter.

The first step on the road to coming to terms with the pain of chronic conditions such as arthritis and soft-tissue rheumatism is to understand what effect they have on your body and why they cause you pain.

The joints

A joint is where two bones meet, and there are a surprising number of different types, which reflect the sorts of work they have to carry out.

Let us start with the simplest, where there are two surfaces in contact, such as one of the finger joints. Here the two bony ends are covered in cartilage – a firm, smooth, gristly tissue which reduces friction. There is also a small amount of fluid in the joint that is secreted by a lining – the synovial membrane – which covers everything inside the joint except the cartilage. Outside the joint is a covering which encloses it completely; this is called the capsule, and it simply separates what is inside from what is outside (see diagram opposite below). Muscles, ligaments and tendons are attached around the joint, helping it to move and keeping it in place. If the cartilage becomes rough, or if the joint fluid decreases, disappears or becomes thick, or the capsule becomes thickened, or the tendons moving the joint stiffen up, the joint will become difficult to move and probably painful as well.

In a more complicated joint, more problems can arise. A few of the different types will illustrate this. The hip joint is a 'ball-and-socket' joint, where

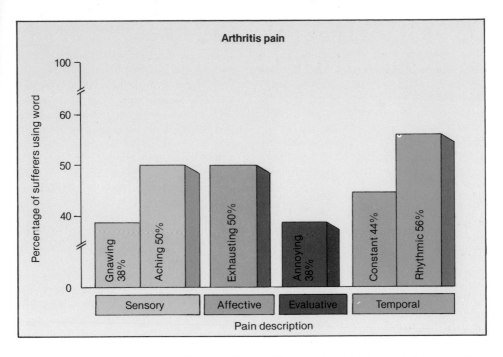

The most commonly used words from the McGill Questionnaire (page 18) to describe arthritic pain.

The anatomy of the finger joint (right) and a knee (left).

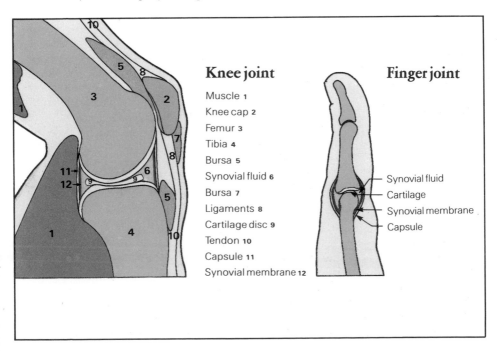

Knee joint

Muscle 1
Knee cap 2
Femur 3
Tibia 4
Bursa 5
Synovial fluid 6
Bursa 7
Ligaments 8
Cartilage disc 9
Tendon 10
Capsule 11
Synovial membrane 12

Finger joint

Synovial fluid
Cartilage
Synovial membrane
Capsule

the top of the thigh bone – the femur – fits into a hole in the pelvic girdle. The shoulder joint also has one bone (the humerus) which has a ball, but the socket part (the scapula) is very shallow and the ball only rests on it, held in place by ligaments and muscles. This joint, because it is less restricted by bone, has a wider range of movement than the hip joint. The latter has to be very solid and relatively rigid to take our weight; the shoulder does not bear weight but has to be able to move the arm in all directions.

The elbow joint, although with a more limited range than the shoulder, can flex and extend the lower arm and can also rotate the hand. The wrist, like the foot, is made up of a group of small bones with joints in between, each moving a little. If you consider the combination of possible movements that can be made by the shoulder, elbow, wrist and fingers working together, all of which adds up to arm activity, it is possible to understand the disruption which can occur when one or more of these joints cannot perform its normal movement.

These movements depend on the muscles around a joint contracting and pulling on the bones of the joint. At the end of each muscle, there is a tendon which is attached to the bone. These tendons are very close to the capsules of some joints, and to save wear and tear by friction and to absorb shocks, flat bags of fluid called bursas are placed between the two. These fluid containers have different shapes, depending on which joints they are protecting. For instance, where the tendons going to the fingers pass over the wrists, they are encircled by bursas which are long, thin tubes, whereas in the shoulder, a bursa cups the outside of the joint. Some joints have more than one bursa. The knee, for example, has fifteen.

There is another way that the prob-lem of friction is reduced, and a good example of this is in the knee joint. Here the thigh bone forms the upper part of the joint and the shin bone or tibia the lower part. The thigh bone is attached to the shin bone by a tendon which passes over the front of the joint. However, if it remained as it was, this tendon would soon wear out from use, and to avoid this, the part of the tendon at the front has become bone – the knee cap (the patella). There is another fea-ture of the knee joint which is of par-ticular interest. Because of the weight that has to be taken on this joint, its centre is reinforced and lubricated by separate pieces of cartilage which al-most fill the spaces between the two bones. The same arrangement occurs in the jaw where similar high pressures develop in the joint during chewing.

The rheumatic diseases

There are four main types of rheumatic disease, which can affect almost all of the joints and muscles of the body.

Osteoarthritis This condition is also called osteoarthrosis. If the cartilage and fluid within a joint are not effective in preventing wear and tear, the carti-lage breaks down and becomes rough, and the bone is exposed. The part of the bone near the joint gets thicker and the joint becomes stiff, while the two ends of bone grind together painfully. This pain can vary from a dull ache to an excruciating pain on movement. This type of rheumatic disease is mainly degenerative, that is, there is a constant wearing away of the cartilage.

Osteoarthritis accounts for about 60 per cent of all rheumatic diseases, and over 80 per cent of all people over the age of fifty-five show some joint changes due to it. Women are much more likely to suffer from this condi-tion than men, and it tends to appear at the 'change of life' – a woman's menopause – when the female hormones are decreasing. The joints most commonly affected are those which are most likely to suffer wear and tear, such as those of the hands, which explains the swollen knobbly hands seen in many older women. The same thing does occur in men but at a later age, although this wear and tear may be aggravated and so can occur at an even earlier age, as happened in the following example with one of my patients.

Joe came to see me, complaining of pain in his right arm. When I examined him, I found that the pain was actually concentrated in his right shoulder. The left one was perfectly normal but it was difficult for him to move the other one in almost any direction. He obviously had osteoarthritis with some inflammation present as well, and this puzzled me since Joe was only forty-three years old and osteoarthritis usually develops in people over fifty. However, it turned out that Joe was a house painter and had spent much of his life wielding a brush with his right hand. In effect, the age of his good left arm was forty-three but his right was really about twice as old because of the extra use he had given it. It was not surprising that an eighty-six-year-old shoulder joint was giving trouble!

The problem was to persuade Joe to switch his paint brush from his right to his left hand. There was no other way to deal with his problem. Needless to say, he eventually did this but not without much complaint about how the quality of his work was suffering. I very hard-heartedly told him that his work was not suffering half as much as his right shoulder would be if he went on using it in the old way. Joe's case illustrates one effective method of treatment: if you cannot change the patient, see if you can change the conditions. It can work well, and I will be discussing this in more detail later.

Osteoarthritis is also more common in joints which have had an injury in the past – a joint at the ends of a previously broken bone or a joint which had been dislocated – but mostly it is old age which does the damage, merely because, the longer you live, the more likely it is that you will have suffered some damage to the joints. It seems to be the penalty of old age, and may account for the fact that more women suffer from it than men, since women live longer. In particular, it is the reason we slow up, and the more joints that are affected, the more the slowing-up occurs. The constant ache on moving is most distressing and not good for the temper either.

One of the characteristic features of the pain of osteoarthritis is that it is worse on rest. This is obvious in the knees, when sitting down for up to an hour will aggravate the pain so much that you have to get up and walk around the room. You will also find that the affected joint or joints are very stiff in the morning when you get out of bed, and it may take some time to get moving in the morning – to get rid of the stiffness.

You might think that exercise would help but, in fact, too much activity also makes the pain worse. 'Too much activity' does not mean what is normally regarded as a regular programme of exercise – this type of movement is vital to prevent the joints from stiffening (see pages 30–3) – but rather exceeding the amount of exercise that you are capable of, given the amount of disability and pain you may have.

Frank, for instance, was not very pleased with me when I was unable to control his pain so that he could do the three-mile walk he had taken every morning of his life until increasing pain had gradually reduced it. The fact that he was seventy years old and getting increasingly stiff cut no ice with him. He complained that one of the great pleasures of his life had been removed. Unfortunately, his moving parts required a complete refit, and medicine at the moment does not allow for this – yet. However, the development of 'new part' surgery progresses steadily – new hips, knees, shoulders and elbows are all available but, with the exception of the artificial hip, none approaches the performance of the real thing. Luckily, with treatment (see later in the chapter) Frank was still able to get out and about relatively free of pain, although not as much as he had when he was younger. It was simply a question of accepting and adapting to the changes that come with age.

The common sites of rheumatoid arthritis.

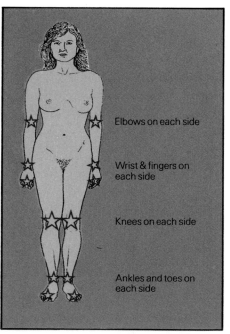

Elbows on each side

Wrist & fingers on each side

Knees on each side

Ankles and toes on each side

Rheumatoid arthritis occurs in about 2 to 3 per cent of the population and is three times more common in women than in men. Most people who have the condition are aged between forty and sixty. When the synovial membrane (see page 25) lining a joint becomes inflamed, the joint can become damaged. Unlike osteoarthritis which affects perhaps one or more different joints, in rheumatoid arthritis, the same joints on both sides of the body are involved – both hands, both ankles and so on.

The inflammation particularly affects the joints of the hands, arms and legs, which are swollen, stiff and painful on movement. This is worse on waking in the morning, and it takes you some time to get going – just like those with osteoarthritis but worse. Rheumatoid arthritis may not be confined to the joints but can affect the whole body. You may have pain, tenderness and swelling of major joints such as the shoulders and knees, as well as stiffness and swelling of the finger joints, and this can be combined with fever, anaemia (a lack of iron in the blood) and depression. In fact, the depression may be one of the two most obvious features, the other being loss of movement with pain.

The cause of this inflammation is not understood. It may be due to an unusual virus infection or it may be caused by an upset in your body's defence system when, for some reason, your antibodies, which are supposed to protect against outside invaders such as bacteria, turn against the body itself.

On average, the course of the illness lasts for several months and leaves some disability behind, usually unstable joints, among other things, although around 45 per cent of sufferers recover completely. It is very much the exception for it to progress to the stage of crippling (only about one sufferer in ten is severely disabled), but it often stops and starts up again. It is not known what causes these remissions or why the disease does not always recur. Research is being conducted into this to see if the remissions can be brought on by medical methods.

Gout is one of the commonest diseases of the joints, mainly affecting men over the age of forty. It is caused by an alteration in the body's chemistry, in which uric acid, one of the body's waste products, accumulates in the body and forms crystals. When the crystals form in the joints, gout occurs. A tendency to have high levels of uric acid in the blood is often inherited, and the joints that are most usually affected are the elbows, knuckles, knees or toes. In fact, gout of the big toe accounts for over 75 per cent of cases.

Gout comes on fairly rapidly, perhaps waking you up during the night with a red, swollen and agonizingly painful joint. The pain can be so bad that you cannot bear to have even bed sheets touching the inflamed area. Resist your first impulse to take a couple of aspirin, because this drug can slow down excretion of uric acid from the body. The best first-aid treatment is to apply hot or cold compresses to the joint. Arrange to see your doctor at the first possible opportunity, and he or she may prescribe drugs that are highly successful in relieving symptoms, including the pain, and preventing further attacks.

Sometimes gout strikes only once, but without treatment it usually recurs. It can be triggered off by losing weight, by overeating and drinking or by eating certain types of rich food. So to help avoid attacks, don't indulge in excesses of alcohol or food, and steer clear of heavy beers, red wines and port, as well as foods high in uric acid, such as fish roes and offal.

Soft-tissue rheumatism, or fibrositis, are general terms used to describe the aches, pain and tenderness of muscles, ligaments and tendons which generally follow a strain or tear. This is then followed by inflammation which prolongs healing. One particularly common type of soft-tissue rheumatism is 'tennis elbow', which is caused by small tears in the muscles which join together the upper and lower parts of the arm. It can often develop during a hard game of tennis, but is also a result of the hard playing of other sports as well as other activities.

Usually rest and the taking of a painkiller such as aspirin are all that are needed for treatment, and the pain and other symptoms will gradually subside. If this does not work, then other methods will have to be tried, such as heat treatment (Chapter 12), exercise (overleaf) and the use of other anti-inflammatory drugs and injections to the painful area.

The common sites of gout.

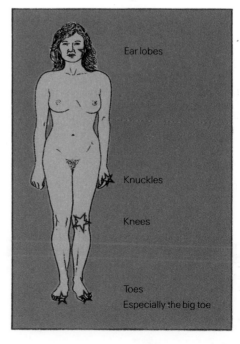

Ear lobes

Knuckles

Knees

Toes
Especially the big toe

Other rheumatic conditions In addition to the above four types, there are many rheumatic conditions which are mixtures of several of these. Thus there can be combinations of wear-and-tear and inflammation occurring together, or first one and then the other. There are also some diseases which start with an infection and are then followed by joint disease, such as occurs in rheumatic fever. Pain can also happen when the bursas in the joints become inflamed – a condition known as bursitis or, more commonly, 'housemaid's knee' when it occurs in that joint. Treatment for this is similar for that of soft-tissue rheumatism.

How the pain can be reduced

The treatment of the rheumatic diseases is carried out over a long period and does not 'cure' any of the conditions, except soft-tissue rheumatism. But it will make you feel better and enable you to move more freely, as well as preventing further pain and disability.

Medical treatment

Drugs Various drugs are used to reduce the inflammation, and thus the pain and swelling of both osteoarthritis and rheumatoid arthritis. The most common – *and* the most effective – is aspirin (see page 92), but others such as indomethacin, naproxen and fenoprofen are also useful.

Corticosteroids (commonly called steroids) such as cortisone are remarkably successful in reducing the signs of inflammation in the joints. But, unfortunately, because of their side-effects they cannot be taken on a long-term basis. However, for temporary relief in some instances, these may be used.

Gold injections are sometimes given to those with rheumatoid arthritis: these are given in courses lasting at least twenty weeks, and in two-thirds of patients they gradually relieve inflammation and may switch off the disease.

Surgery is, unfortunately, not a cure-all, but the replacement of arthritic hips by plastic or metal joints is nowadays very effective. There are also knee, ankle, shoulder, elbow, wrist and finger joint replacements, but the outcome for all of these has not been nearly as good as for hips and intensive research is still going on.

Sometimes the swollen synovial membrane that lines an affected joint will be removed, but this gives relief for only a year or two.

Rest and exercise

While the pain of a rheumatic disease or joint injury is at its strongest, 'acute' stage, it is important not to overwork your body, including your joints. Resting in a chair or, if the illness is more serious, in bed or even in hospital is crucial at first, so that you do no more damage to your joints and/or muscles.

When the acute stage has subsided, you should try to move all your joints through their full range of movement every day or even two or three times a day. By this I do not mean that a painful joint should be forced through this normal range; but as far as it reasonably can, each joint should be moved so that it does not get stiff and form adhesions (membranes that stick together) inside it merely because of disuse.

Medical doctors, medical osteopaths and physiotherapists will first demonstrate a programme of gentle movement and then you can carry on at home. If extra vigorous movement or manipulation is needed, it should be done under their supervision. The following exercises, illustrated on pages 32–5, are some examples from such a programme. Starting slowly, do a few of these at a time, and gradually increase the number you can perform as your body begins to respond to treatment. In addition, other gentle activity, such as walking (especially on grass, which is not as hard on joints as hard surfaces are), should be carried out little by little – see also Chapter 12.

Neck and head exercises The neck is affected by a whole host of conditions from injury such as whiplash to the rheumatic diseases, but the following movements are relatively easy to carry out (see page 32). First, turn your head as far to the right as is comfortably possible and then to the left. Do not rush from one side to the other, but take your time. Next, look up as far above your head as possible, trying to point your chin at the ceiling – you can't, but that gives you the idea. Follow this by placing your chin on your chest – remembering to keep your mouth shut. Finally, lean your head and neck sideways to the right, trying to put your ear against your shoulder (which is impossible). Then do the same on the left side. Repeat all these movements as many times as you can comfortably, up to a maximum of ten.

Shoulder and arm exercises To put your shoulder joint through a full range of its movement, start off with your arm by your side (see page 33). Then raise it forwards until it is horizontal. Then continue until it is straight up above your head, and then put your hand behind your neck. Then slowly lower your arm to your side again and put your hand on the small of your back as high up as it will easily go. These movements can be repeated as many times as is comfortable up to ten.

Finger and hand exercises Movement of the hands and fingers is enormously important, not only gross movements such as making a fist, but also fine movements such as are in-volved in picking up a piece of paper or a knife and fork (or chopsticks). Using a piece of paper is a good exercise to improve these finer movements (see page 34): pick it up, crush it, roll it between both hands, tear it (which means holding it). To help the mobility of the joints of the hands, touch each fingertip to the thumb in turn.

Spine and back exercises See page 52.

Leg exercises These exercises are done while you are lying on your back (see page 35). First, raise one leg, keeping the knee stiff. Then try to touch your abdomen with your thigh, bending your knee at the same time. This is repeated with the other leg.

If the leg is weak, this type of movement may not be possible but the knee can be exercised by swinging the lower leg while you sit in a chair. Other leg exercises can be done using weights, but for this, expert help is required. There are many exercises for particular joints and groups of joints and there is not room to mention them all here. Further exercises can be found in *Overcoming Arthritis* by Dr Frank Dudley Hart. However, I hope that I have said enough for you to realize that it is not dangerous to exercise if you suffer from a rheumatic disease, provided that this is not very painful and not carried to excess. If in doubt, do discuss it with a professional.

Learning to cope with rheumatic pain
As I have already mentioned, people do not all feel pain in the same way, and having a high or low tolerance of pain can make all the difference when it comes to coping with the pain of a chronic rheumatic disease such as osteoarthritis or rheumatoid arthritis. Your frame of mind is of the utmost importance: if you are positive and op-timistic, the pain will not seem nearly

Head and neck exercises   1a & b: Slowly turn head first to right, then to left. Increase repetitions as they become easier.

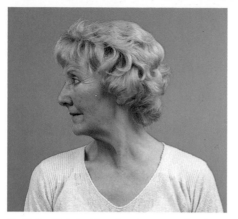 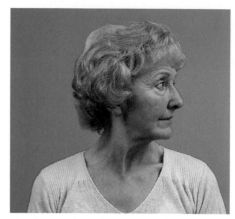

2a & b: Point chin slowly upwards, then point it down, tucked into neck. Keep shoulders level.   3a & b: Slowly tilt head first to the right, then the left as far as is comfortable. Keep shoulders level.

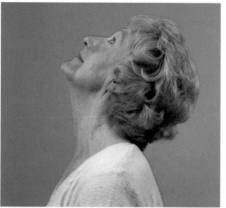 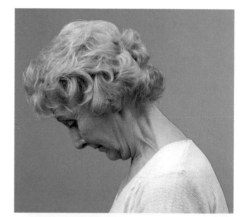

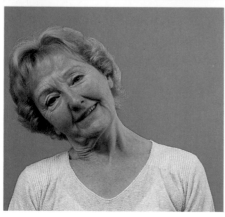 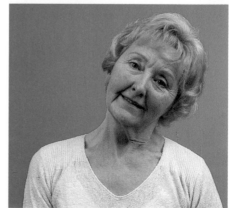

Shoulder and arm exercises Starting with arms by your side, lift one arm straight up in front of you. Lower hand to back of neck, or lower if you can. Drop arm to your side and bend it up behind back. Repeat with other arm.

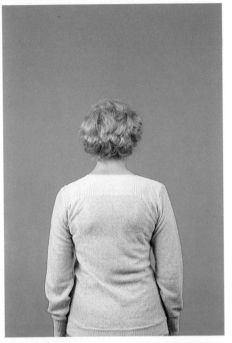 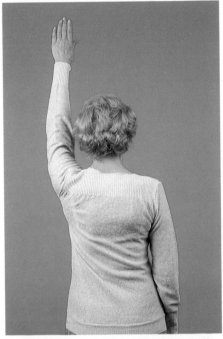

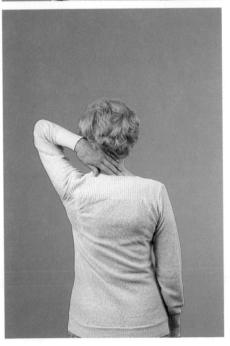 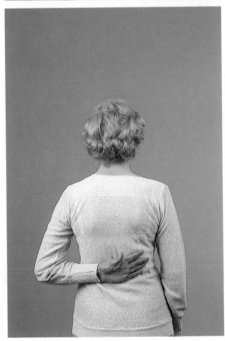

Hand and finger exercises   1a & b: Slowly crush a sheet of paper into a tight ball.

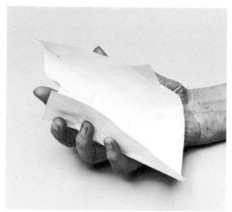 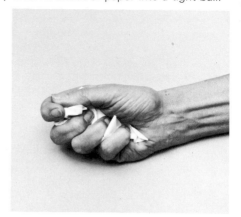

1c & d: Spread paper out with fingertips. Tearing paper is another good exercise.

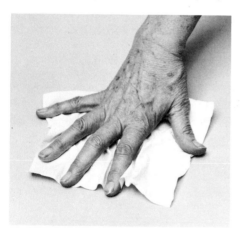 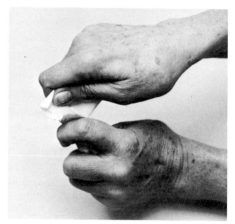

2a & b: Make a circle with thumb and little finger, then slowly slide thumb down to base of finger. Repeat with each finger.

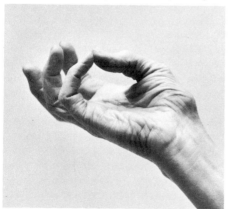 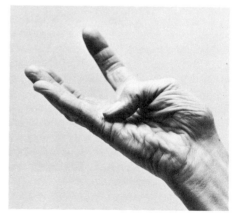

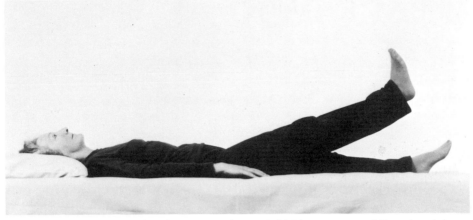

Slowly raise leg to an angle of not more than 45°. Hold to a count of five, then bring knee towards chest. Lower slowly and repeat with other leg.

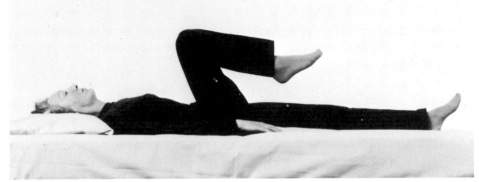

as much of a burden as if you are negative and pessimistic. Many of the mental mechanisms to avoid feeling pain discussed in Chapter 2 will be of help to you – particularly occupying your mind with something else, be it knitting, watching television, gardening, reading or running a business.

On the practical side, there are many specially designed devices that can be bought – such as tap turners and teapot tippers – that can make daily life easier. Some simple home modifications like replacing door knobs with lever handles and electric switches with cord pulls will conserve your energy *and* your temper! Like my patient, Joe, you

may find that you will have to alter some of the ways in which you do things, but in exchange for some awkwardness and irritation, you will find that your daily activities are easier to do. A great deal of help can be obtained from occupational therapists, who will give advice on adapting yourself to some of these activities, and will also help you to retrain your arms and legs to make certain movements, to enable you to carry on as normally as possible.

Other useful methods of pain relief – relaxation, heat treatment, massage and 'rubs', acupuncture – which could well be of help, are described in the final two chapters of this book.

4. BACK PAIN

All pain is a result of alterations in the human body, be it from a chemical burn, a crushed finger or an alteration in the general anatomy of the body. In the latter, a part of the body has changed shape, as in an arthritic joint, and this produces pain through distortion. Pain in the back has much to do with this, and can vary from a mild throbbing ache to excruciating stabbing agony that can equal or exceed the pain of cancer (see diagram on page 19). The Arthritis and Rheumatism Council estimate that in Britain alone 20 million working days a year are lost because of back pain, and the figures are comparable in other Western countries. Of course, this statistic does not take into account the millions of people who are not employed, or those who continue to work despite the pain. Back pain seems to affect both sexes equally, around half the patients seeking help for it from their family doctor being women.

Anatomy of the spine

'The back' is a very loose description of an area which, to the medical profession, starts where the head is connected to the spine and goes all the way down to our 'tail' (see page 38). Most people think of the back as not including the neck, while many think of it as only comprising the area from the waist down to the tail. To avoid confusion, the following terms will be used: the 'cervical region', which comprises the part of the spine in the neck; the 'lumbar region', from the waist downwards; the 'low back', the lower half of the lumbar region together with the mass of bone below it, known as the sacrum; and the 'thoracic region', that part of the back to which your ribs are connected.

Because the head is quite heavy and moves easily, there are a number of ways in which pain can develop at the head–neck junction. In addition, each part of the spine has a potential for pain due to the shape and function of its bones, and particular pains may occur because of the special movements required at each level.

Your spine is made up of building-block bones called vertebrae which are placed one on top of the other, giving you the ability to stand upright and protecting the vital spinal cord which they surround. The spine must be flexible so that bending and stretching are possible yet, at the same time, it must provide a solid base in three places: the junction of the head and neck (the cervical region); the junction of the ribs and spine (the thoracic region); and the weight-bearing lumbar region.

The head and neck (the cervical region) The first of these crucial points is where the head is attached to the top of the spine by the two uppermost vertebrae which are much thicker, flatter and stronger than the other five cervical vertebrae in the neck. The highest vertebra supports the weight and allows nodding movements. While the second

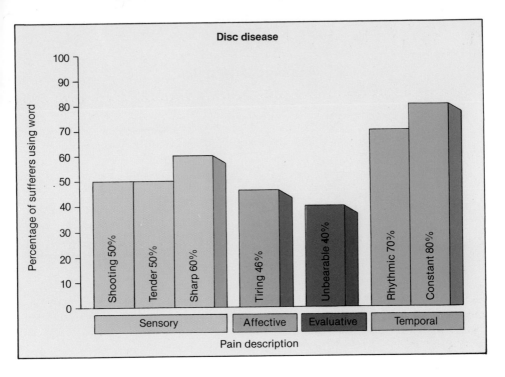

The most commonly used words from the McGill Questionnaire (page 18) to describe the pain of disc disease (page 44).

provides a swivel which allows the head to rotate. Naturally, both these joints are subject to tremendous wear and tear and can become arthritic and painful. In addition, they – and the ligaments which surround them – are particularly prone to damage during accidents when the heavy head may be tossed around, as in a whiplash injury (discussed later). Rotation of the head is also affected if you develop a 'stiff neck'. You cannot rotate your head, and if you want to look sideways, you have to move the whole upper part of your body.

In addition to the nodding and turning functions of the two top vertebrae, further movement is supplied by the cervical vertebrae below them. These allow a certain amount of sliding of one vertebra on another, enabling the neck to bend forwards, backwards and to each side.

The ribs and the spine (the thoracic region) This is the part from which the chest wall is suspended. It is in this region that the heart and lungs are located and where breathing takes place. There are special joints on each side of the vertebrae where the ribs are attached, while the other ends of the ribs are joined to the breast bone (sternum) at the front of the chest. When you breathe in, the ribs move sideways and upwards, carrying the breast bone with them. In this way, the size of the chest increases and your lungs have to expand to fill the extra space. The thoracic vertebrae have to provide the rigid platform from which this movement takes place, and therefore this part of the spine cannot move very much. Being the most stable part of the spine, it is far less frequently the source of pain as the top and bottom sections.

Anatomy of the spine

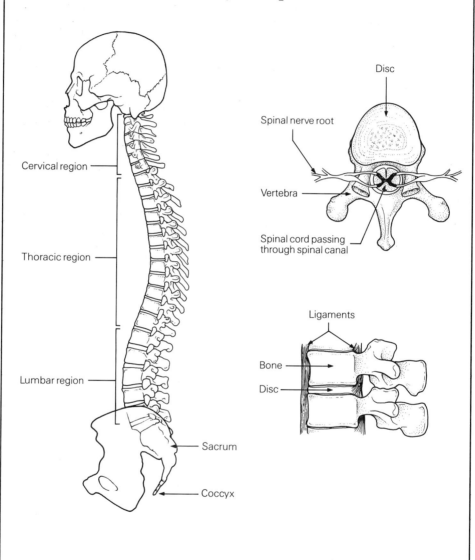

Cervical region

Thoracic region

Lumbar region

Sacrum

Coccyx

Disc

Spinal nerve root

Vertebra

Spinal cord passing through spinal canal

Ligaments

Bone

Disc

The bottom of the spine (the lumbar region) This is the weight-bearing part of the spine which transmits the whole weight of the upper body on to the pelvis and then on to the legs. Because of the relatively enormous load, this part of the spine frequently goes wrong, and the types and problems of pain that are produced here are numerous. This pain is generally referred to as 'lumbago'.

This portion of the spine, plus where it fits on to the pelvis, is known as the lumbosacral region. The upper part consists of the five lumbar vertebrae which are distinguished by their size and thick bone: they get larger as they get lower, in other words, as they carry more weight. The sacrum, a large mass of bone, fits underneath the lumbar vertebrae and, through this, the weight is taken to the pelvis. To do this, the sacrum lies at an angle to the vertebrae and also to the pelvis. It is attached to each by joints and ligaments, and be-cause of the angles, there is enormous strain at the upper and lower ends.

Below the sacrum lie five very small vertebrae which together are called the coccyx, connected by a joint and liga-ments to the sacrum. The coccyx is the last remnant of our tail, and its only importance is that, if this joint is dam-aged, it can produce a rather unpleasant type of pain on sitting.

The vertebrae Each vertebra has four joints called posterior facet joints – one on each side above and one on each side below – which connect the verte-brae to each other. There are also the special joints in the thoracic region which are connected to the ribs. All of these joints can be strained by direct injury such as a whiplash injury to the cervical region, by injury caused by lifting too heavy or awkward a weight, or by inflammation as in a rheumatic disease such as arthritis (discussed in Chapter 3).

A vertebra's four posterior facet joints – two above and two below. These are freely supplied with nerve endings.

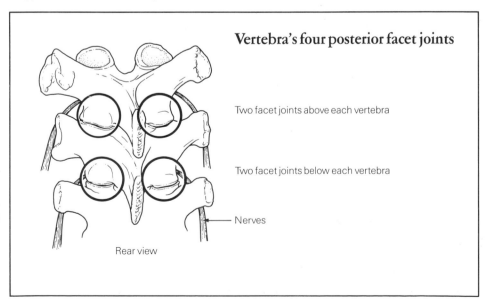

Vertebra's four posterior facet joints

Two facet joints above each vertebra

Two facet joints below each vertebra

Nerves

Rear view

One of the features of the facet joints is that they are supplied freely with nerve endings which come from not one but several of the nearby nerves. Thus when pain develops from these joints, it may appear to come from a widespread area or may be quite local, that is, from quite a specific place.

In and around all the vertebrae of the spine are strong muscles and ligaments which both help the vertebrae to move and keep them in place. Any strain or tear in these can cause considerable pain.

Discs are of supreme importance in the efficient and effective working of the spine as a whole. They are twenty-three flat pieces of cartilage – tough, gristly tissue – placed between each vertebra, and they provide a certain amount of give and, to some extent, act as shock absorbers. They are, in fact, very complicated pieces of body equipment, and as we get older, they deteriorate so that some of their function is lost. This and the actual alteration of the joints of the spine make us much stiffer as we get older.

The disc tissue is not the same consistency throughout, as its centre tends to be more fluid and under a higher pressure than the outer rim. In the lumbar region, where the whole body weight is pressing downwards, the discs are much larger than in the neck and also have much greater semi-fluid centres. These centres act like large ball-bearings between the vertebrae. The discs are not a passive portion of the spine but are absolutely necessary to its proper functioning.

When the edge of a disc weakens, the softer centre may push out through the weakened section and produce pain by pressing on a nerve in the spinal cord. This is what happens in disc disease, more commonly (but inaccurately) called a 'slipped disc' (see pages 44–8).

The spinal cord Finally, brief mention should be made of the most important structure of the spine, namely, the spinal cord. This is the nerve structure which runs from the brain down the spine through the protective arches of bone of the vertebrae, and is also protected by the muscles and ligaments which surround the spine. Our nerves arise from the spinal cord and make their way between the bones and muscles to other parts of the body. If they are affected in any way – by injury, pressure or infection – pain can be produced. Not only that but the pain may be 'referred' – that is, it is produced in the spine but it feels as if it comes from somewhere else (see pages 12–13). This is how a damaged lumbar disc can produce pain down the leg.

Pain in and around the spine

The vast majority of pains around the back – using the term 'back' to mean from the back of the head to the end of the coccyx – are not serious ones, but by that I mean that they are not dangerous to life – they are certainly most uncomfortable and sometimes very disabling for a time. About 99 per cent of back pain is due to mechanical problems, either to injury or to wear and tear.

As you get older, your body does not repair itself as well as it did when you were younger, and your ligaments and muscles are not as flexible. Thus it is easy to strain a joint if it is already partly damaged because of degeneration. Fortunately, most of these mechanically produced pains are relatively easy to deal with, and only about 1 per cent of all back pains need serious treatment.

'How bad is the pain?' is the question that everybody asks and nobody can answer accurately. As I said earlier, no two people experience pain in the same way. The pain is what you say it is. If you have ricked your neck, the

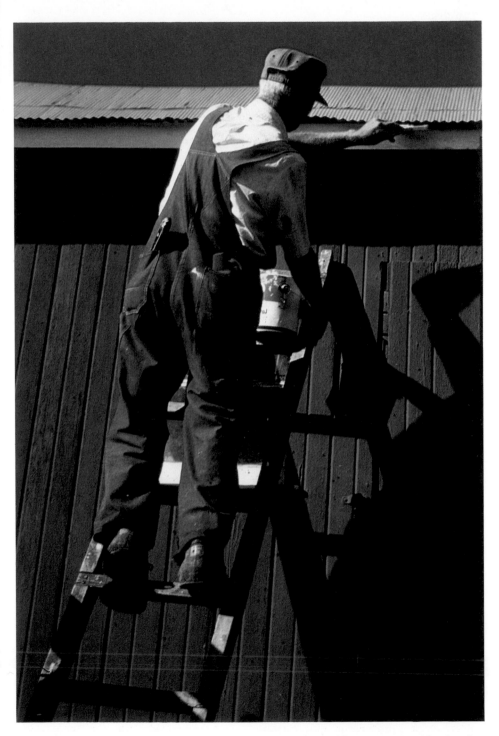

Staying in an awkward position for a long time can trigger off an episode of back pain.

pain and stiffness may stop *you* from working for a day, but if the same thing happens to your next-door neighbour, he may have to go to bed for a week, while Bob down the street would hardly notice it.

It is not always necessary to have an outside injury to your back in order to feel pain. It can be triggered by straining or just by staying in an awkward position for some length of time. You have probably tried your hand at painting a ceiling, and I expect will remember the stiff neck that you had at the end of it. You had been looking up at the ceiling with your head thrown back for some hours, and this is a position which puts the small joints, muscles and tendons in the neck under strain. The result is discomfort which lasts for some days, going from a pain to a stiffness and then disappearing. If you repeat the performance, there will be another episode of pain which will last longer and disappear more slowly.

This, in fact, is one of the lessons to be learned about spinal pains: do not repeat the cause of the injury too soon. Before you do, work up to it by gradually increasing your efforts over days or even weeks, using gentle exercise that increases in strength and range before putting the affected part under strain again. I shall be examining this idea again later in the chapter and be giving suitable exercises.

Diagnosing back pain

While most back pains are caused by no more than the strains of daily life and are relieved by rest and gentle exercise, others – resulting from more dramatic as well as everyday injuries and from disease – need more specific diagnosis and treatment.

A syndrome is a pattern of symptoms (what the person feels) and signs (what the doctor looks for) that a patient has, and discovering this pattern leads to the diagnosis of what is wrong

with him or her. For example, if you fall over, are then in great pain with your arm bent in an unnatural way, you can safely make the diagnosis of a broken arm. The combination of fall, pain and bent arm is a syndrome, albeit a very simple one.

In exactly the same way, syndromes can be described for the painful conditions around the spine. The structures in and near the spine are limited to muscles, ligaments, bones, nerves and the spinal cord itself. (Blood vessels – arteries and veins – are also present but play a less prominent role.) It is quite easy to understand that when a muscle, a ligament and a section of bone are near each other, the nerve supply to each is much the same, and therefore no matter which tissue is damaged, any pain will appear to come from the same part of the body. The basic symptoms will be the same.

It is at this stage that a doctor will want to know about other features of the condition, such as 'Did it come on slowly or suddenly?', 'Did you hear or feel a clunk when it happened?', 'Is it painful all the time or only when you move in a certain way?', and so on. After the questions come the tests: 'Bend this way, then that. Does this start up your pain?', 'What happens when I press here?', and so forth. Usually these questions are enough, but occasionally, in some conditions, medical tests and possibly X-rays have to be carried out. Once the diagnosis has been made, treatment can begin.

The common causes of pain in the back

Sudden pains in the back are the result of damage somewhere in the spinal tissues which arises relatively quickly. The following are the most common causes:

Inflammation This type of pain develops slowly but steadily throughout the day, and is not helped by resting. It is usually due to the small joints in the spine – the facet joints – becoming inflamed. This does not mean that they are 'infected' but that they have been damaged in some way so that they have begun to repair themselves. Often this is a prelude to the development of osteoarthritis (see pages 26–8).

The first stage of the repairing process is inflammation, when there is swelling of the tissues and the production of fluid. This means that the capsule surrounding the joint becomes thicker and stiffer, does not move easily and is painful. In the neck often only one joint is affected, while in the lower, lumbar region, more than one is common.

Locked joints These are often caused by the spine having been twisted. The pain may occur suddenly and you know immediately that the movement you have just made was the cause. A locked joint will be painful all the time, but the pain becomes more intense when you move. You may find that there are certain movements that you must not make otherwise one of your joints will lock. Although this is most common in the knee, some of the facet joints of the spine can become locked by the two bony halves of the joint jamming or sticking together; and usually you find it more difficult to straighten up than to bend down. In all joints there is a small quantity of fluid between the joint surfaces which acts as a lubricant. If this gets squeezed out from between the joint surfaces by the twisting action, the joint is more likely to lock. This type of locking tends to occur at the spinal end of the rib joints in the central, thoracic region as well as in the facet joints.

Once a joint has jammed you can try very gentle movements to unlock it. If this does not work or is too painful, the correct manipulation carried out by a qualified osteopath (see page 54) or an injection of fluid into the joint may sort out the problem.

Tears Muscle, ligaments and tendons can be torn because of a sudden or awkward movement, and this produces immediate pain. A true tear in any of these is very rare, though, and in fact, rather than tearing, it is more usual for the end of a tendon to tear away from the bone to which it is attached, along with a small flake of bone. In other words, it is the bone which gives way and not the tendon. It all depends on the amount of force used and on the health of the tendon, as often there has been previous damage over a prolonged period before a tendon will tear away from a bone. When a muscle or ligament tears, there is a 'knotting' of it which can be felt and seen as a lump under the skin. It is immediately intensely painful and this is increased whenever it is called into activity again.

Tears usually occur after a lot of previous strenuous muscle use and trauma – particularly in sportsmen and women. The Achilles tendon, which runs down behind your ankle to your heel, is the commonest site of injury. These tears respond to rest and gentle exercise, which will be discussed later in this chapter.

Faulty posture and spinal abnormalities Perhaps the most common cause of backache is faulty posture when sitting, and this may be increased when reading or typing for prolonged periods. Long-distance driving can also produce pain in the upper spine, when the head is fixed in one position for long periods of time. I have already mentioned painting a ceiling, but sitting at an angle to a television screen is just as potent a cause of a painful ricked neck.

Incorrect posture when standing can

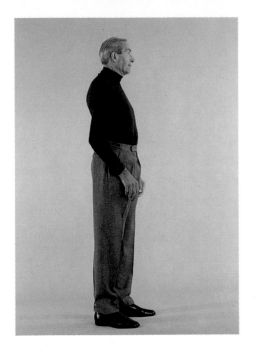

Good posture.

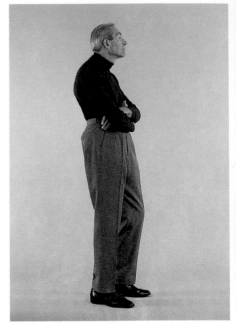

Bad posture.

also produce backache. Learn to stand tall and distribute your weight equally on both feet. Avoid standing with the weight on only one leg, but if you must, then alternate the weight-bearing leg. One good – and traditional – test to see if you are standing properly is to balance a book on the top of your head. If you sag or bend in the wrong way, the book falls off!

There are also some minor abnormalities of posture due to an exaggerated curvature of the spine. A round back (kyphosis), a hollow back (lordosis) and the condition called scoliosis, when the spine (looking at it from the back) curves first to one side and then the other, often produce minor aches in the muscles under strain, although just as often there is no pain at all. The spine curves normally, and if this is exaggerated or reduced, then mild pain can result. If you have one leg even slightly shorter than another – about one in four of us do – this can also put your spine under stress. Any-

one with these types of curvature should be especially careful to stand tall and to sit properly. In addition, exercises to strengthen the back muscles will help (see page 52).

Finally, there are some conditions where a part of a vertebra is not completely formed of bone or it is injured, say, by jarring, and it slips, stretching the ligaments and sometimes causing pain. This is called spondylolisthesis, and occasionally a surgical operation is needed to fuse together the affected vertebra. Just as often, though, symptoms are very mild and disappear, or do not occur at all.

These are some of the common causes of pain around the spine. I shall now go on to consider more specific conditions in some detail.

Disc disease
What is commonly called a 'slipped disc' is the most common cause of severe pain in the back. Around 1 person

in 200 is affected in a year, two-thirds of the total number being men. The pain usually comes on quite suddenly, but it may also arise as a soreness which gradually becomes worse over a few hours so that it is almost impossible to move freely. In fact, some movements cannot be done at all and lying down in bed is the only thing you can do. When there, you cannot get up in the usual way, and it may be necessary to roll over on to one side and lever yourself up, while your legs slide over the side of the bed as you sit up. Bed is the best place if you suffer from this type of pain.

The pain is produced by the soft centre of a disc breaking through the outer layers and pressing a finger of tissue on the nearest nerve. This is called a disc protrusion. Inflammation and swelling of the surrounding tissues rapidly result, accounting for the rapid increase in pain. Resting for a few days helps this swelling (called oedema) to go down and, with it, the severe pain subsides. Occasionally a disc will suddenly go back into place, in which case the pain disappears as quickly as it came. You usually know when this has happened, feeling it as a click or as if 'something just went back', just as you often know that something came out just before the pain started. Disc disease may be caused by lifting a weight in a rather awkward position.

This is what happened to Jim, one of my patients: 'I was unloading a lawnmower from the back of my car. This has a fixed tail-gate, so I first had to lift the mower over the car's end. It was a cumbersome piece of equipment, and although I could manage the weight well enough, it was awkward. I knew I should have waited for another person to equalize the lift, but I was impatient and did it myself. I managed quite successfully, but as I put it on the ground,

I felt something "go" in my back and I was immediately struck by a pain which shot through my back and down my left leg. Having placed the mower on the ground, I found that I could not straighten up, and I was stuck in that position until my wife and son arrived and helped me into the house. Eventually I recovered enough to make the effort to get to bed.

'In due course, my doctor arrived and diagnosed a slipped disc – which everybody including me had diagnosed as well! – and prescribed at least four days' bed-rest. In the end, I was actually in bed for two weeks and it was another week before I was able to return to work.'

This is not an unusual story. It was not the first time that Jim had had an episode of back pain, but all the others had cleared up in a day or two and he had managed to carry on until he worked it off.

Pain from a disc pressing on the spinal nerve in the lower back can be referred down the back of the leg.

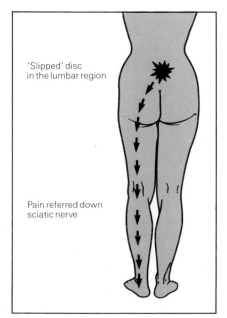

'Slipped' disc in the lumbar region

Pain referred down sciatic nerve

As I have already mentioned, there are discs between each two vertebrae and so it is possible to have a slipped disc at any level of the spine. That is the theory, but in practice, there are only two places where discs get pushed out frequently: the lumbar region and the cervical region – in other words, at the top and bottom of the spine. The reason for this is that both places are where the most movement takes place: turning, twisting and bending. Furthermore, the lumbar spine supports the weight of the upper body.

Where the pain is felt When a disc is pushed out, it can press on the surrounding tissues enough to cause a spread-out, constant, severe pain or ache in either the neck or the lower, lumbar back. However, when the disc presses on the spinal nerve which is nearest to it, pain is also felt in the area which that nerve serves – in other words, the pain is referred to that area (see page 45). This means that, in the lumbar region, the pain can be referred, as it did with Jim, down the back of the leg as a form of sciatica, because it is carried from the spinal cord by the sciatic nerve, the largest in the body. While in the neck it can be referred down the arm by the brachial nerves. In the leg, it may actually get as far as the foot and toes, and in the arm, it may be referred to the hand and fingers. The sensation may not always be completely painful. There may be tingling or pins-and-needles as well as pain. It all depends on how much pressure the disc produces, and whether the process is in the early stage, when pain is more likely if the disc pushes out suddenly. If it is clearing up or is developing slowly, tingling is more probable.

Diagnosis of disc disease Because a disc presses on a nerve, it stops the nerve from working properly, and this is also shown by the alteration in the nerve reflexes. There are two reflexes in which doctors are especially interested when considering lumbar disc problems: the knee jerk, when the foot gives a little kick or jerk forward when the knee underneath the knee cap is tapped with a doctor's hammer; and the ankle jerk, when a similar movement of the foot occurs – in this case, downwards towards the floor – when the big tendon above the heel is tapped. As the pain down the leg has a special pattern, depending on which nerve is affected, discovering this pattern by finding out which reflexes are not working properly can be useful in deciding which disc has 'slipped'. Finally, as these are 'mixed' nerves – that is, they carry both power nerves to the muscles and sensation nerves to the skin – the identification of the weakness of certain muscles and the numbness of certain parts of the skin is also used in finding the abnormal disc.

When it is suspected that you have disc disease, your doctor will first ask you how the pain started and whether there have been any previous attacks like this. The position of the pain and the state of your reflexes will be assessed, then a note will be made of how you feel a pinprick and a light touch (checked with a piece of cotton wool). When all these facts have been assembled, a fairly accurate idea of the presence of a disc protrusion can be made and at which level of the spine it has occurred.

Non-surgical treatment of disc disease Your treatment will be based on whether your damaged disc is a new one or one that has happened before. If it is recent or if it recurs only at long intervals, bed-rest, heat treatment (see Chapter 12) and painkillers (see Chapter 10) will be prescribed for at least three weeks. Around 90 per cent of those experiencing the pain of disc disease for the first time will recover after three weeks of simple bed-rest.

Sometimes after the first, extremely painful – or acute – stage of a disc protrusion, manipulation by an osteopath may enable the protruded portion of the disc to slip back into position (see page 54). Before that happens, traction may help to relieve the pain. This is a method which uses your own weight to pull the vertebrae slightly apart, and thus relieve the pressure on the nerve from the swelling which, in turn, reduces the pain. Your legs are attached to the foot of the bed which is then raised so that your weight tends to slide to the bed head and the pressure on the disc is relieved. It is also possible to fit patients into machines which, by means of harnesses, provide a controlled but stronger pull for a shorter time. These are to be found in hospitals and physiotherapy departments, and should only be used when skilled help is available.

If this treatment is successful, one of two things happens: the disc protrusion decreases and no longer presses against the nerve root, or the nerve root slips sideways away from the protruded disc and thus reduces the pressure. In either case, the pain diminishes markedly and eventually disappears completely, and you can then return to normal activity.

There is one type of disc protrusion which needs very quick treatment. Any condition which causes difficulty in passing urine calls for medical attention, but this is doubly important when a disc is suspected, as it implies that a large piece of disc is pressing on the nerves controlling bladder action. If this is not dealt with quickly, there may be long-term bladder difficulty. Sometimes it is the bowel that is involved but, fortunately, both conditions are relatively rare.

What can be done if initial treatment is not successful? It is usually pos-

sible to make most diagnoses of disc protrusion on the basis of the clinical history – that is, what the patient tells the doctor – and then the condition can be treated as above. What should be done, though, in the relatively rare instance of there being no improvement in, say, three weeks? There are a number of possibilities and each is the preference of some physicians, so it is impossible for me to state what others would do. When a diagnosis has been arrived at and treatment for three weeks has not been successful, I prefer to have a special type of X-ray investigation called a radiculography carried out. In this, a water-soluble dye is injected into the fluid surrounding the spinal cord (called cerebrospinal fluid or CSF). The dye spreads throughout the fluid inside the sheaths surrounding the nerve roots, and if one of these nerve roots is pressed upon by a disc, the sheath is closed off and the CSF cannot get into it. The dye is radio-opaque, which means that it stops X-rays, and thus when an X-ray is taken, instead of the normal appearance showing dye in the sheaths, there is nothing there at all – further evidence that a disc is present. Sometimes the disc is so large that it presses on other things and this, too, may be seen, and other conditions which involve pressure on nerves may show up as well. One of the benefits of using a modern water-soluble X-ray dye is that it is absorbed into the blood after a few hours and then excreted from the body in the urine so none of it remains in the spine and it cannot do any damage. In fact, if there is any doubt about the result of the X-ray, it can be repeated again safely.

There are other types of X-rays which use radio-opaque dyes injected into other places. For instance, they can be injected directly into the disc itself and this will show if the outer rim of the disc is broken and if part of it is protruding. The dye can also be injected into the veins near the spinal cord and this will show up any distortion from a different angle. They all have different values, and some doctors favour one type of X-ray over another because they are more expert at interpreting it or performing it.

The very modern CAT scan X-rays can show up much more detail and are used when available – sometimes in place of the dye method. CAT scanning is the preferred procedure in the United States.

Surgery When a disc does not get better through bed-rest, heat treatment, painkillers and traction; when it has recurred several times; if there is chronic pain; or bladder or bowel function has been impaired, surgery may be the next course. Any operation on the spine is a major one and there are complications which can occur, so surgery is not entered into lightly, and in any case, only 1 in 1,000 of those suffering from backache require surgery.

The operation – called a laminectomy – involves the complete removal of the offending disc, via a small opening in the spine. To avoid the formation of a disc made up of scar tissue which can be as painful as the damaged one that has been removed, many surgeons fuse the bone on each side of the removed disc. To do a fusion takes a little longer, there is a little more risk, there may be more pain after the operation and there are other factors to take into account before this is performed. In addition, since movement of this part of the spine is now impossible, this means that more stress is placed on the joints and vertebrae around it which can, in turn, make them more vulnerable to further damage.

After a simple disc protrusion has been removed, it is the usual treatment in our unit at Liverpool for patients to be kept in bed for only two or three days. While in bed they can lie in any position that is comfortable for them (they usually choose to lie on their sides), although they will find it difficult to move without help for the first day or so. Physiotherapy is started on the first day after the operation. By the third day they are able to sit out of bed for short intervals and many begin to walk with help on the fifth. This is when back exercises are begun to strengthen these muscles.

Normally these patients will be ready to be discharged from hospital after ten days or so, but they are asked not to return to normal activity until six weeks or more have passed. Even then, they are warned against straining their backs by such things as lifting heavy objects in a stooping position, crouching for any length of time or jumping from a height. Apart from these sensible precautions, the vast majority return to an active and normal life very quickly.

Cervical and lumbar spondylosis
Spondylosis is a disease of the older person, and it has been estimated that half of those over the age of fifty and three-quarters over sixty-five suffer from it. In this condition, there is a progressive deterioration in the cervical and lumbar vertebrae – those near the top and bottom ends of the spine. This, in turn, can affect the facet joints which hold the spine together, with thickening of the vertebral edges, hardening of other bony surfaces and a reduction in the spaces in which the discs lie. The undue wear and tear affecting the joints can then spread to neighbouring soft tissues. The disease may confine itself to bones and joints, or it may spread to produce pressure on, or irritation of, the spinal nerves. Unlike osteoarthritis with which it is frequently confused (see Chapter 3), the pain of spondylosis is intermittent and responds well to rest. It is also possible for you to find

some position of comfort.

The cause of this disease is little understood, although damage, bone abnormalities and joint diseases such as rheumatoid arthritis tend to start it off. It is most likely that the disease starts in the discs, and once these have begun to degenerate, the condition spreads. It is not always possible to distinguish cervical spondylosis from cervical disc disease, although disc disease can occur in an otherwise normal spine, and the two conditions often occur together.

Treatment with a collar I have already mentioned that there is a lot of movement in the cervical (neck) portion of the spine so it is not surprising that, when there is chronic irritation around the cervical joints, the movement of those joints will produce pain in the neck and often down the arms, sometimes causing headache from the neck up to the top of the head. This pain is reduced by preventing the movement of the joints and this is why the muscles in the neck go into spasm – that is, they contract and tighten up – Nature's way of reducing movement. The muscles at the back of the neck are much larger and stronger than those at the front and sides, and the spasm in them is therefore much more noticeable. Unfortunately, after a time, the muscles themselves start to become painful because of the damaging effect of the constant contraction.

Treatment of this type of cervical pain can often be helped by the wearing of a cervical collar, which limits movement and supports the weight of the head, allowing the neck muscles to relax. These collars may be prescribed by your family doctor or a specialist, and range from soft ones which limit the larger movements to very stiff solid ones which hold the head and neck completely rigid. If it helps, you should wear your collar whenever your neck is in pain; if it makes no differ-

A surgical collar limits painful neck movement.

A corset gives support for lumbar spondylosis.

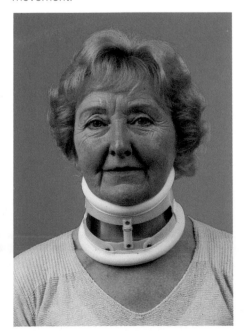

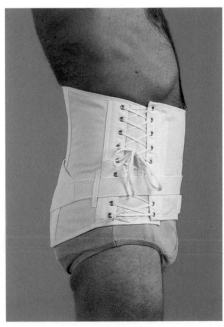

ence, leave it off. Luckily, although the pain can be quite acute to start with, it usually settles down in a few weeks.

Treatment with a corset The corresponding condition in the lumbar region is produced by essentially the same process, but because of the great problem of weight-bearing, it is almost always associated with disc disease. The main exception is where direct injury to the lumbar facet joints may produce the condition without disc disease. Just as cervical spondylosis can be relieved by a collar, so in the lumbar region an orthopaedic corset may be used. These are stiff and very firm, with the object of providing solid support, and may be prescribed by an orthopaedic surgeon or a neurosurgeon. The advice I have just given for when to wear a collar holds good for corsets also, but neither corsets nor collars should be worn for more than six weeks and, instead, gentle exercises should be performed to strengthen the muscles to provide support.

Other treatments may be used to relieve the pain of both cervical and lumbar spondylosis. First, you might be given an injection of a mixture of local anaesthetic and a long-lasting anti-inflammatory steroid drug into the joint to see if this relieves the pain and lack of movement. The procedure will either be carried out in your family doctor's or specialist's surgery, or in hospital under X-ray control. In many cases, a simple injection of this type will result in weeks or even months of relief. When the irritation and pain settles, gentle exercises (see pages 54–5), massage (pages 110–111), traction and painkillers can be used to prevent a recurrence.

Whiplash injuries
There are other situations in which the spine's facet joints are likely to be affec-

ted. Car accidents are a potent cause of injury, and a whiplash injury in the cervical region can be produced in a driver or passenger when the car in which they are sitting is hit from behind by another car. The neck of the person in the front car is first thrown back and then forward, and the bones, joints, muscles and ligaments of the neck are stretched very quickly, first in one direction and then in the other, often becoming strained and painful.

This is just what happened to Louisa: 'I was driving away from doing my weekly shopping when my car was hit violently from behind by another. I was a bit shaken up but I was able to deal with the problem of the accident and got my own car to the garage. About an hour or so later, I noticed that my neck was sore, and I was woken up in the night by intense pain at the back of my neck where it joined my skull. I could hardly turn my head, and the pain then spread up over the back of my head and down my neck.'

Louisa had X-rays done after the accident, and fortunately no fracture was discovered. Her pain was severe for a few days but gradually subsided, being considerably helped by a cervical collar, which she could not bear to wear at first because of the tenderness. I saw her a couple of months later and she still had some tenderness and limitation of movement. An injection like that given for spondylosis (see previously) into her upper facet joints combined with another in the small muscles and ligaments at the base of the skull made a great difference. Eventually, the pain and stiffness settled down over the next three months.

I was told a somewhat similar story by Kevin, whose car was hit by another coming out of a side road: 'My pain began a few hours after the accident, and I felt it on one side of my back and just above my backside. Oddly enough, it was on the side furthest away from where my car was hit that I had the worst pain, as if I had had a sudden twisting wrench to my lower spine. My pain lasted for many months and people thought I was either malingering or neurotic.' Far from imagining or faking his pain, when Kevin was examined it was found that his injury had occurred in the lumbosacral region. The area over his sacroiliac joint in his buttocks and one of his lower lumbar facet joints on the same side were extremely tender, and these were given injections on a number of occasions which helped a great deal.

Nerve pain in the neck and head

Called suboccipital neuralgia, this not uncommon pain in the upper neck and the back of the head is a neuralgia (literally, 'nerve pain') of the greater occipital nerve, which extends over your skin and scalp from the second cervical vertebrae upwards to most of the back half of your head, spreading as far as the back of your ears. It tends to occur in older people, but can affect the younger age group, especially after whiplash injury (see previous section). There is usually tenderness in this area of the scalp, and when you move your head, there is considerable pain. Sometimes this may spread forward and feel like a pain behind the eyes.

This syndrome is well known, but doctors usually do not find any abnormality in the vertebrae or the soft tissues. Nevertheless, when this type of pain occurs, your doctor may well decide to have skull and neck X-rays taken, particularly to make sure that there is no inborn abnormality of the head/neck junction.

Treatment To treat this condition,

the wearing of a cervical collar will probably be recommended for up to a month, and the immobilization of the head and neck that results may settle the pain and neuralgia. An injection of a local anaesthetic (such as that used for spondylosis, see opposite) into the greater occipital nerve may be tried to see if the pain is relieved and, if it is, a semi-permanent solution can be injected at a later date to provide long-lasting relief. This will numb all or part of the area of skin where the pain is usually present, and many sufferers prefer this to the pain, although it can be a weird sensation to place the back of your head on a pillow and not feel the pillow on the back of your head. As in other forms of back pain, heat treatment, acupuncture, electrical stimulation and other simple measures can also be tried (see Chapters 11 and 12).

Rheumatic nodules

One of the most common causes of pain in the neck and back of the head and in the lower back is the presence of nodules. These are small lumps in muscle, which can be felt quite distinctly and which are extremely tender. Not only that, but because they cause spasm and pain in the muscle fibres in which they are located, the whole of that muscle and others near it become tender and, on occasion, extremely painful. The pain can be referred (see page 12) along the nerves near the nodule. So, if the nodule has affected the muscles around the shoulders, the pain may be referred to the point of the shoulder, to the part of the neck nearby and sometimes as high as the back of the head. Similarly, the pain can be referred down an arm.

There are two places in the body where nodules tend to form: the area at the top of each shoulder, and lower down at the junction of the loin and

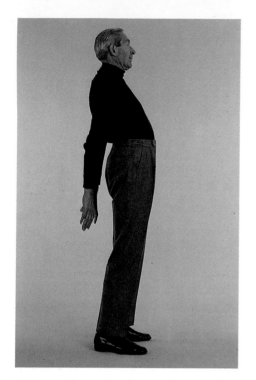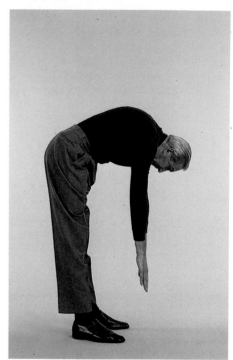

Mid- and lower-back exercises 1. Bend slowly backwards as far as you comfortably can. 2. Slowly bring yourself upright and bend forward towards your toes as far as is comfortable. Repeat.

Spine muscle exercise Lift up head and shoulders as far as you can manage comfortably. Hold to a count of five. Rest and repeat.

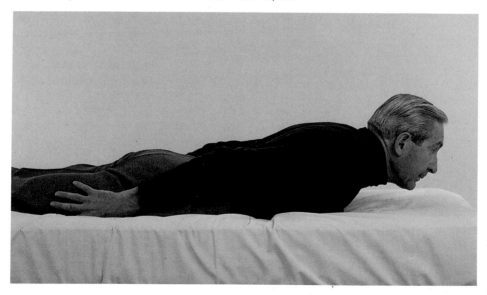

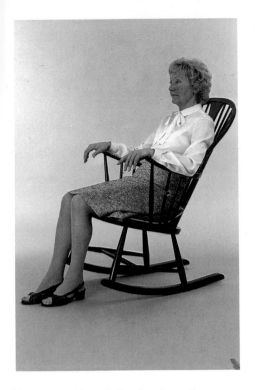

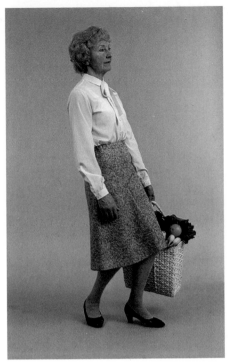

Using a rocking chair stimulates the nerves, helping to block the painful sensation of backache.

To avoid damaging your back it's important when lifting heavy weights to bend your knees and keep your back straight.

buttock at the hip girdle. The likely cause of both kinds is the same – physical injury – as these two areas contain the muscles that are most active in, respectively, moving the arm, and tilting the pelvis and lifting the leg; and they are most likely to get strains as well as small areas of muscle damage during your working life. After this damage occurs, a small scar is formed and this is where nodules tend to develop.

Treatment of painful nodules is simple. In the early stages, rest, massage and heat treatment (see Chapter 12) are usually enough to provide good relief. In later stages, when the nodule has become large and very tender with local and referred pain, an injection of local

anaesthetic into it usually settles the pain, and since the pain immediately disappears when the correct nodule has been injected, there is no doubt about the diagnosis or its correct treatment. Often a small amount of a long-lasting steroid solution is injected at the same time, as this tends to speed healing and prevent recurrence.

Anne, one of my patients, was unfortunate enough to have fallen heavily on to her back from a step ladder while decorating her home. She suffered heavy bruising with bleeding beneath the skin of her back. As expected, when she eventually got over this and the rest of her injuries, she had many scars in the muscles below the bruised area. As a result, nodules developed and over a period of time these were injected and they disappeared, only for another group of nodules to appear later. Although the nodules recur every so often, it is possible to treat them fairly easily, and Anne has been able to lead a full and satisfactory life.

Treating back pain

Suggestions have been given for the treatment of particular kinds of back conditions, but there are a number of general measures which are employed for most of them.

When back pain first occurs, the best thing to do immediately is to make the back as immobile as possible through bed-rest. Total rest, though, is often impossible because every movement – even coughing and sneezing – is painful, and so you should take a painkiller such as aspirin or paracetamol (acetaminophen in the United States) to control or ease the pain and discomfort. Sometimes doctors will also prescribe tranquillizers or sedatives to help you get some rest. When inflammation is part of the problem, you might be given a non-steroidal anti-inflammatory drug, such as indomethacin, although aspirin also has this property.

Manipulation A gentle massage is one form of manipulation and this is discussed in more detail in Chapter 12. The kinds of manipulations performed by trained manipulative therapists and physiotherapists include massage and exercises which stretch muscles and put joints through a full range of movements, as well as rhythmic, repetitive movements to persuade a joint to move properly. Only when a joint refuses to improve using the above techniques does a manipulative therapist use a specific thrusting movement to release it,

repeating this occasionally to prevent it from stiffening up again.

The best way to choose a manipulative therapist is by his or her reputation. Always be sure that whoever you chose has the proper qualifications and is a member of the relevant professional association which will have a strict code of conduct.

Other methods of treatment – acupuncture, electrical stimulation, heat treatment and so on – are discussed in Chapters 11 and 12. Finally, one excellent habit to adopt is to use a rocking chair, which not only exercises the back muscles, but also stimulates the nerves in the skin to help block painful impulses.

Exercise

Once the acute stage has passed, you should start moving your muscles – at first only a little, then more as you heal. A physiotherapist may have to help, or your family or friends can be taught how to move you through some simple, passive exercises. Once your doctor thinks you are well enough, you can begin some gentle active exercises – preferably in consultation with him or her, or a physiotherapist – to help regain some or all of the movement you have lost. Which exercises you do will depend on your own level of health and fitness. If this is not too bad, then it will be possible to go through all the movements slowly that are described opposite and illustrated on page 52. If pain limits movement, then the range, too, must be limited, and if an exercise brings on pain, you should stop immediately. Do not exercise until it hurts. The exercises should be done slowly and carefully, putting your joints through as full a range of movement as you are able. In this way you can often perform effective movements that would be too painful if done quickly.

Another tip to remember is for bending forward from the waist. While some people have always been flexible enough to touch their toes, there are some of us who have never been able to do this, and if you cannot do this when you are healthy, there is no point in attempting it when you are recovering from injury or disease. So, instead of trying to touch your toes, try to touch your kneecaps instead, gripping your thighs above your knees if you like in order to help you get up again.

To stretch the neck (cervical) muscles See page 32.

To stretch the mid- and lower-back muscles Standing upright, bend back as far as you can go, then raise yourself upright again. Now reach forward as far towards your toes as you can go comfortably (see page 52). Repeat up to ten times.

Another exercise to help the same regions is again done standing upright. First bend to the right, letting your arms hang loosely by your sides; return to an upright position and then bend to the left. Repeat as often as is comfortable, up to a maximum of ten times.

To strengthen the spine muscles Lying face downwards, place your hands down beside your body and then lift your head and shoulders half as far as you can if you strain. Hold this for a few seconds, then rest and repeat up to six times on the first day, gradually building up the number of lifts to twenty (see page 52).

Other exercises for the back can be found in *The Back: Relief from Pain* by Dr Alan Stoddard, also in this series. Exercising in water – hydrotherapy – can also be useful under the supervision of a physiotherapist, as the water will hold you up, thus relieving the pressure on your spine. Heated water itself can be very comforting.

Preventing back pain

Do
- If necessary, lift heavy weights with knees bent and your spine straight, balancing the load equally in both hands.
- Stand erect and ensure that all working surfaces are at a comfortable height.
- Have a firm but comfortable mattress which supports your spine. A board under your mattress provides a firm base.
- Use chairs which support the spine and allow both feet to be flat on the floor.
- Have a car with seats that give support to the back and neck and which can be entered easily – without having to bend double.
- Go on a diet if you are overweight. The extra weight puts added stress on your back.

Do not
- Stand in a fixed position for too long. When ironing, cooking, washing up, and so on, change your position repeatedly, sit down and walk around.
- Lift heavy weights with your back bent.
- Suddenly twist or jerk your back, or overexert your back by doing work or exercise you are not used to.
- Sit in easy chairs which make you slump.
- Sleep in a soft bed which encourages the curve of the spine to sag.
- Walk or run on hard ground or concrete paths. Stay on the grass when possible and run or jog on your toes.

5. PAIN IN THE CIRCULATION SYSTEM

The effects of faulty circulation

There are three important varieties of pain which may occur in the circulation system – and all are termed 'vascular' pain, vascular meaning 'of blood vessels'. The first and the most important of these is cardiac pain (that is, in the heart), next is pain in the foot and leg, and thirdly there is pain in the arm and hand.

All of these arise because the circulation in the heart, leg and arm has been somehow affected for the worse. In all cases when this happens, either the blood supply to parts of the organ or limb is just good enough to keep them alive but is not sufficient to get rid of the waste products of muscular activity, so that activity has to be reduced; or the blood supply is so faulty that parts of the organ or limb become damaged or may die.

The heart pumps the blood around your body through the blood vessels. The blood carries oxygen *to* the tissues via the arteries, and waste products *away* from them via the veins. These waste products are produced by all the different tissues in the body, and if they accumulate in excessive quantities, they can poison you. They are normally washed out of the tissues into the bloodstream, through which they travel until they are excreted by the kidneys and, to some extent, the bowels and the lungs. If the blood circulation of any part of the body becomes so poor that it cannot remove the poisons, then some of the tissues in that area will be damaged or will die until what is left can be kept alive by the diminished circulation.

Clogging of the arteries: atherosclerosis

An artery is made up of three layers. There is a relatively loose outer layer which carries nerves and small blood vessels, as the artery itself has to have a blood supply. Next is the thickest layer which is composed of elastic and muscle tissues, and enables the artery to contract and expand in response to the needs of the part of the body it supplies. The innermost layer, or intima, is a thin, smooth lining which is designed to allow the blood to slip past it without any hindrance.

The blood contains a number of different constituents such as the red and white cells, and the platelets. These last are small cells which stick to each other when part of the body is damaged – as when you are cut or when the intima of an artery becomes rough. When the platelets become sticky, this starts a process which causes blood to clot, and so it is very important that the insides of the arteries (and the veins, for that matter) remain smooth, otherwise they may become blocked by blood clot.

The condition called atherosclerosis causes the intima of arteries to become thickened and rough, and this is very often the starting point of most coronary thromboses (heart attacks) and arterial obstructions (blockages of arteries) in the leg and arm. About 80 per cent of all adult heart disease in the Western world is caused by atherosclerosis.

What causes it? There are a number of reasons for the high incidence of atherosclerosis, and not all are fully understood. The Western diet contains far too much fat in foods such as dairy products, red meat and oil, and it is also over rich in cholesterol, found mainly in eggs, liver and saturated fats like butter. It is now generally accepted that these two may have a bad effect on the blood chemistry. In addition, most people do not take enough exercise to keep themselves in good health, and too many people smoke cigarettes, which can cause, among other problems, contraction of the arteries with a consequent reduction in blood flow and an increase in blood pressure. All these things put added strain on the circulation system. There is also some evidence that the stress of modern life may have something to do with the developing of heart disease. For more details about the factors which may cause heart and other artery disease, see *Beat Heart Disease!* by Dr Risteard Mulcahy, in this series. What is important to realize is that atherosclerosis of the arteries can produce irreversible changes and pain in the organs which are supplied by those blood vessels.

Heart disease

Heart disease occurs when one or more arteries supplying the heart muscle gradually become thickened, reducing the space in which the blood travels, and the blood supply to that area of the heart is reduced. If a clot forms, lodges in the narrowed coronary artery and blocks off the blood supply to a section of the heart, this is called a coronary thrombosis, or heart attack. (I shall be describing this later on in the chapter.) If the narrowing continues gradually, a stage is reached when a part of the

heart muscle has a good enough blood supply when you are at rest, but it is insufficient when you become active, say when you walk around. This results in pain called angina.

Angina, or angina pectoris, to give it its full name, means simply 'pain in the chest'. It is a common condition, usually occuring after the age of thirty in men, and later in life in women.

Angina may also come on more subtly than I have described. For instance, you may be all right walking about on flat ground but the circulation to the heart may not be able to keep up with the extra pumping necessary when you walk up an incline or up stairs. The blood supply may also not be enough if you become excited or eat a heavy meal – in fact, after doing anything that makes the heart beat faster. During physical activity, the pumping

When an artery's intima, or inner lining, becomes rough, a blood clot will form and may eventually block the artery.

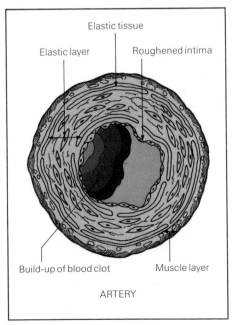

Elastic tissue

Elastic layer

Roughened intima

Build-up of blood clot

Muscle layer

ARTERY

of the heart muscle produces waste products in such quantities that, in an area of the heart with damaged arteries, the blood supply cannot take them away. As they increase, they begin to affect the heart muscle, and this is felt as pain. The pain of angina is severe, is felt in the centre of your chest, and usually lasts only a few minutes. If you keep on with your activity, the pain will become more severe and will spread – usually into the left shoulder and arm (sometimes into the right), and possibly up the neck and into the jaw. On rare occasions, it may not be felt in the usual places but may occur in the abdomen or jaw first (see 'Referred pain', page 12).

Usually the pain is so strong that you must stop and rest wherever you are. Larry, one of my patients, is one of these unfortunate sufferers: 'The last time I felt this pain, it was so intense and filled me with such fear that I had to stop in the middle of a busy road while I was crossing it, despite all the cars that were rushing past me. Only when the pain disappeared could I again move slowly to the sidewalk to rest there.'

You can recognize angina by its occurring in the following sequence: physical exertion, pain, rest, relief. But having a pain in the area of the heart can be misleading, as the cause for it may actually be in the stomach or elsewhere. If you have a pain in this area, you should go to your family doctor as a matter of urgency for a check-up.

Rest is the basic treatment for angina, combined with as much exercise as the heart can manage – in this condition too little exercise is almost as bad as too much. Smoking must be stopped at once. And if you are overweight you should try to lose weight by cutting right down on fatty and high-cholesterol foods (see also page 61).

Sites of angina pain. It usually starts in the centre of the chest and spreads leftwards. Sometimes it can arise on the right side and move to the right arm.

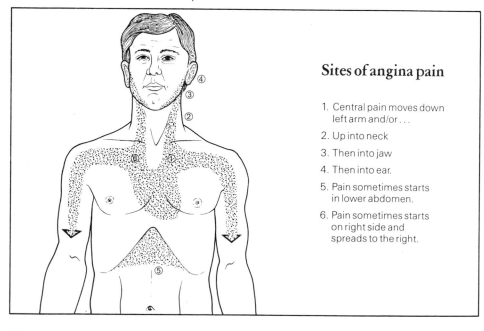

Sites of angina pain

1. Central pain moves down left arm and/or . . .
2. Up into neck
3. Then into jaw
4. Then into ear.
5. Pain sometimes starts in lower abdomen.
6. Pain sometimes starts on right side and spreads to the right.

Certain drugs can also be prescribed to control the pain of angina: vasodilators, which expand the blood vessels around the damaged ones so that these carry more blood, taking the load off the diseased ones; and beta-blockers, which block the action of adrenaline (epinephrine), produced by the body as a response to emotion and exercise, and which acts on the heart.

A minority of angina sufferers may also benefit from an operation which replaces damaged arteries with healthy ones taken from elsewhere in the body.

Heart attack Around ½ million people every year in Britain have a heart attack, or coronary thrombosis, and at least two-thirds of this number survive the attack. Many heart attack victims have previously suffered from angina, and, as with angina, we have to look at the blood supply to the heart to understand the causes of the condition.

Between them, the right and left coronary arteries carry all the blood from the circulation to the heart muscle. If one of these becomes blocked, some of the heart muscle must inevitably die, and if enough of this happens, the heart stops pumping properly and then may stop altogether.

Each coronary artery has branches, these branches also have branches and so on. What damage is done depends on at what stage of the branching the blockage occurs. To some extent, there is a certain amount of connection between the smaller arteries so that, if one gets blocked, a supply of blood can be obtained from another and little or no damage results. The larger the arteries involved, the less likely it is that this alternative blood supply will develop.

When an artery becomes blocked in this way, it is usually due to atherosclerosis that has roughened the inner lining and has gradually reduced the diameter of the artery. This process is followed by a clot forming, and when this completely blocks the artery, a coronary thrombosis is the result.

Pain in the chest is the commonest symptom of coronary heart disease, but it does not always occur, and from time to time doctors see patients with massive and dangerous coronary thromboses without pain. The pain of a heart attack can build up from an indigestion-type of pain behind the breast bone into an intense, heavy pain in the chest. Or it can come on suddenly and you may not be able to get your breath, feel very afraid and faint if you are standing, because your blood pressure has fallen. As with angina, the pain may spread into the shoulders, arms, jaw, neck, abdomen and back. There will also be sweating, restlessness and pallor. Unlike the short-lived pain of angina, coronary thrombosis pain may last for several days before gradually disappearing. If severe, this pain is usually alleviated by being given the narcotic pain-killer morphine (see page 93) until the acute stage has passed.

In about 80 per cent of acute coronary (heart) attacks, the heart muscle that has been affected will die after about an hour and then can no longer help in the heart's pumping action. It forms what is called an 'infarct' (a segment of dead tissue), and if this is not too large, the heart action can continue – with some difficulty – and you recover. What happens depends partly on the size of the infarct and where it is, and partly on the state of the heart muscle to begin with. For example, have you had a previous coronary thrombosis? Do you have high blood pressure? Have you taken regular exercise? Did your heart have a normal rhythm before the present coronary thrombosis? Fortunately, once most people are helped over the initial danger period, their hearts gradually settle down and return to normal within a few weeks.

59

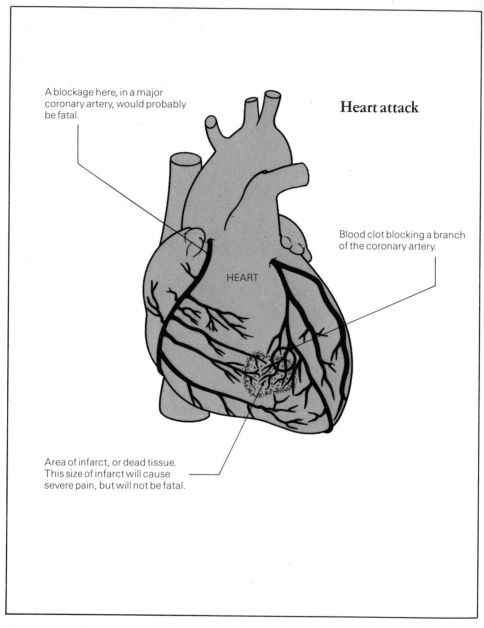

A blockage here, in a major coronary artery, would probably be fatal.

Heart attack

Blood clot blocking a branch of the coronary artery.

HEART

Area of infarct, or dead tissue. This size of infarct will cause severe pain, but will not be fatal.

The results of coronary artery blockage at different levels of the heart.

How to help a heart attack victim If the person's chest pain lasts for ten minutes or more, call the patient's own doctor or get the victim to hospital by ambulance or private car. Stay with him or her and prepare to perform resuscitation if you have been trained how to do it.

How to avoid the pain of heart disease

Adopting the following guidelines will help to prevent you developing heart disease – angina and coronary thrombosis – or to recover from it.

- Lose weight if you are overweight. Your chances of reaching and remaining at a suitable weight are improved if you slim gradually. Although crash diets can achieve results quickly, they are not usually successful in the long term.
- Cut right down on fatty foods, such as butter, cheese, whole milk, cream, oils, red meat and all fried food.
- Cut right down on high-cholesterol foods, such as eggs, liver, shellfish and ice cream.
- Cut right down on salt by not adding it to your cooking or your food at table.
- Increase your intake of high-fibre foods such as wholewheat bread and pasta, wholegrain cereals, beans, and fresh vegetables and fruit.
- In consultation with your doctor – if you already suffer from heart disease – you should try to take some exercise every day. Having heart disease does not mean you should live the life of an invalid. Even walking is good for the circulation. If you want to take up more strenuous forms of exercise like jogging, cycling or swimming, it is very important to take it very easy at first and not to overdo things. Build up to a reasonable level of fitness gradually.
- If you smoke, give it up.
- If you are tense and under pressure, try to reduce the amount of stress in your life. You may find the relaxation exercises in Chapter 12 useful for this.

Atherosclerosis in the leg

Just as the coronary arteries can gradually narrow and eventually become blocked, so the same process can occur in the arteries and their branches in the leg. It is less common, though, for a major artery in the leg to become blocked suddenly and for the blood supply to the limb to cease altogether.

There are a number of major differences between the heart and the lower limbs which are relevant here. For a start, the leg can rest whereas the heart must always keep beating or life is lost. Second, the tissues of the leg are not as specialized as those of the heart and their blood supplies are larger and there is much more in reserve. Finally, portions of the leg can actually die without interfering completely with the ability of the leg to support weight and move the person.

Atherosclerosis of the leg is a common condition, occurring mainly in people over the age of 40. Most likely to get it are those who smoke, are overweight, take little exercise and eat large amounts of animal fat and cholesterol. High blood pressure sometimes is associated with it and diabetes can make it worse. Obviously, the sooner the condition is diagnosed, the sooner treatment can be started.

The results of atherosclerosis of the leg One of the first symptoms may be a cramp-like pain on exercise – what is called intermittent claudication, from the Latin word *claudicare*, 'to limp'. The blood supply of people suffering from this is so poor that the waste products produced by muscular activity are not removed and sufferers can walk only short distances – sometimes only 50 yd (46 m) – before they have to stop because of the pain in their calves (caused by the presence of the waste products). After an interval, when their sluggish bloodstreams eventually remove the wastes, they can walk a bit further before they have to rest again because of the pain. It is a condition very similar to angina, where exercise causes pain in the heart; in claudication, exercise of the leg causes pain in the calf.

Harry is an example of someone who is unfortunate enough to suffer from this: 'I was quite all right until a year or so ago when I noticed that, when I walked a mile, my left calf ached so much that I had to stop walking until the pain went away. If I stopped walking from time to time, as I did when shopping, I did not get any pain. Then, after some months, I noticed the same pain in my right leg, and as time went on, the distance I could walk before the pain came got less and less until it was only a few hundred yards. The pain was now very severe, and if I went on walking, it became worse and worse until I had to stop. After a time the pain would go and I then found I could walk more or less the same distance until the pain returned and the whole process was repeated.'

What can be done? Long before the condition becomes serious, efforts should be made to reverse it, supervised by your doctor. You must stop smoking immediately and, if overweight, must go on a diet. Exercise involving the legs must be taken, even if it is painful, as this will help keep the non-affected blood vessels healthy and may help the affected ones. By using these self-help measures, 90 per cent of those who have suffered from this either improve or suffer no further deterioration.

To relieve the pain of atherosclerosis in the leg, take simple painkillers such as aspirin and paracetamol, and try elevating the affected leg above your hip either by propping your leg up on a footstool, or by lying down and resting your leg against the edge of a chair or the wall, or by raising the foot of the bed several inches off the floor. All these measures will help the circulation through the leg veins. If you get cramp in the leg(s), simply rubbing the affected muscle should help, or you can try a massage technique as described in Chapter 12.

The simplest type of atherosclerosis of the leg to treat is when there is a blockage in only one part of one of the arteries to the leg. This can be discovered by injecting a radio-opaque dye into the artery and taking X-rays showing the progress of the dye through the arteries of the lower limb. Where the dye stops, there is a blockage. The worst problem arises when there is atherosclerosis in many of the leg's arteries and there is a generalized reduction in blood flow throughout the limb.

Other medical treatment can involve any of the following:

- Removing the blocked artery and grafting a piece of artificial artery in its place.
- Injecting chemicals into the artery to increase its diameter and so improve the blood flow.
- Giving drugs which help arteries around the affected one(s) to expand and carry more blood.
- Performing a sympathectomy – an operation in which a nerve that causes the blood vessels to contract is cut.
- There are also some relatively new drugs which may be able to dissolve a clot once it has formed, provided it has done so recently.

Raynaud's disease
This relatively rare disease of the circulation system is particularly common in women but not confined to them, and usually begins when you are in your teens or early twenties. The blood vessels in the arm and hand become so

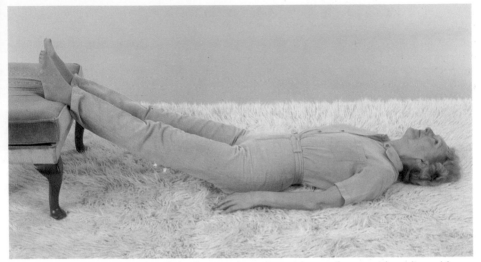

The pain of atherosclerosis of the leg can be relieved by resting your leg above hip level.

sensitive that they are particularly responsive to cold. When the hand is exposed to cold, they contract and reduce the blood supply so that the fingers and hand become blue or white. The fingers become increasingly numb and, after a time, they cannot be felt at all. Later, when you move into a warm place, the tissues of the fingers usually swell up as a reaction to the prolonged contraction of the blood vessels, and the fingers then become red, swollen and stiff. All these stages can give rise to severe, continuous aching pain. When this process continues for years, the vessels can become permanently damaged. Attacks can also be caused by emotion or by vibration, as well as by cold. The treatment of Raynaud's disease is very similar to that of atherosclerosis of the legs. In addition, and most important, the very first treatment is to keep the fingers as warm as possible because, if they become cold, this may start an attack. Thus gloves must always be worn in winter, and there are a few unlucky people who have to wear them in summer as well.

6. MIGRAINE AND HEADACHES

Migraines and headaches involve very different types of pain but are sometimes confused. The reason for this is because both involve pain in the head. Migraine, though, is a condition on its own, with definite stages and symptoms, usually finishing up with a severe headache, whereas headache itself can be produced by many different things, from simple tension to very serious physical ailments, and can vary from mild to severe.

Like back pain, headaches of all varieties are responsible for great losses due to days off work and for the vast amounts spent on pain relief – more than $500 million annually in the United States alone. And it is estimated that one person in three of the Western population has one or more headaches a year.

Migraine

Migraine is a periodic condition in which sometimes very severe headaches are accompanied by a variety of other symptoms. Millions of people throughout the world suffer from migraine. Lewis Carroll, Sigmund Freud and Thomas Jefferson all had it, women fall victim to it three times more often than men, and more than half of all sufferers have their first attacks before the age of twenty and 90 per cent before the age of forty. The word 'migraine' is a corruption of the Latin *hemi-cranium*, or 'half-skull', which describes the one-sided headache that is common in this disorder.

Classical migraine

How you can tell an attack is imminent If you suffer from what is called classical migraine, you usually know when an attack is coming on. You may have a sense of great well-being; you just feel good, better than usual, and this feeling can occur a day or so before the attack. Sometimes you may have a heightened sense of smell or the feeling that you are seeing everything with particular clarity. In fact, any of the senses can be sharpened at this time.

Shortly before the headache arrives, you can have a sensation called an aura, which commonly shows itself as difficulty with or changes in vision. You might have difficulty in focusing or see flashing bright lights, and it is usual for this visual disturbance to progress to loss of some vision; though only very occasionally does this lead to temporary blindness. The aura may also take the form of a peculiar smell, nausea or vomiting. You may lose your voice or the ability to find words, or experience a change in the sensation of touch. Whatever the symptoms, they remain remarkably constant in each attack over long periods of time. The aura normally lasts fifteen to thirty minutes and then begins to fade.

The headache Then comes the headache, which can last from an hour or two to twenty-four or even seventy-two hours. As I have already said, it is usual for it to be present on only one side of the head (on the opposite side to any visual loss or numbness), starting behind or above one eye and then spreading to the back of the head on the same side, or starting in the back and moving forward. The pain can range from a nagging ache to an unbearable thumping and pounding.

During this stage you usually feel nauseated and may vomit, which sometimes will relieve the headache. Some people fall asleep after an attack and wake up feeling normal, but others may be woken up by the headache.

The frequency of attacks is very variable, but up to eight migraines a month is possible. There are a few unfortunate people whose migraine merges into ordinary headaches afterwards and without treatment are never really free of headache at all. However, on average, migraine attacks usually occur once every one to three months.

Common migraine

The principal difference between classical migraine and this variety is that, in common migraine, there are few or no warning symptoms. The first thing that you know is that one of 'those' headaches is starting, and you will then suffer from just as painful a headache as in the classical variety and may vomit or be nauseated before, during or afterwards. As in classical migraine, there is often some relief after the vomiting, and in some people, the attack is over once they are sick. Unfortunately, common migraine can occur more frequently than the classical type – sometimes two or three times a week if you are under stress.

If you suffer with the classical type, you will occasionally get the odd bout of the common type. If you normally get the common type, on the other hand, you will occasionally get an attack of the classical type.

What causes migraine?

Changes in body chemistry People who get migraine seem to have especially sensitive blood vessels under the skin of their faces and scalps and in their brains, which contract when certain chemicals appear in the bloodstream. An attack of migraine is triggered off by the release of these chemicals.

Usually the contraction of the blood vessels starts in the part of the brain which controls sight. That is why one of the first symptoms in classical migraine – the aura – is an alteration in vision, when you may stop seeing in part of your field of vision or may see bright lights or sparks. The contraction of the blood vessels spreads over the brain like a wave. Your vision gradually returns to normal but you feel other things as different parts of your brain become affected. That is why some people get a stiff or numb face, or a sensation of pins and needles down one arm. After the contraction stage, the vessels widen, and most migraine headaches come on at this point.

Trigger factors The reasons why and how these chemicals are released is impossible to say as there are so many things which can start off a migraine attack: stress, not enough or too much sleep, noise, certain smells, excitement, bright or flickering lights. For instance, an attack may be triggered when you are watching the flickering lights at a disco. Other causes are certain foods and drinks (in particular, cheese, citrus fruits, fried food, chocolate, seafood, red wine), changes in daily routine and the weather (for example, hot dry weather, thunderstorms, snowstorms and sandstorms, although the real cause may be a stressful reaction to these conditions). Surprisingly, attacks do not usually occur *during* a period of stress but only *after* that stress is over.

65

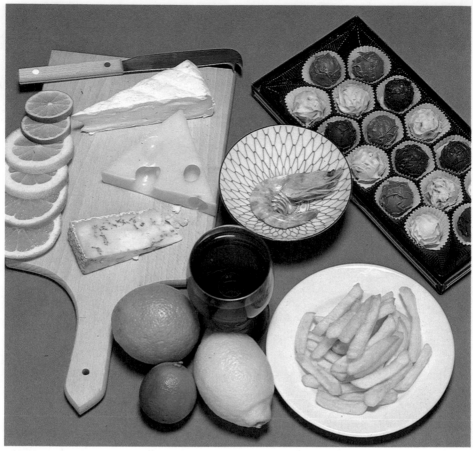

Cheese, seafood, red wine, chocolate, citrus fruits and fried food can all trigger off a migraine attack.

Hormones and the Pill Migraine and other types of headache are about three times more common in women than in men, but this imbalance only occurs from the age of eleven (when girls tend to start having periods). It appears that a drop in the circulating amount of one of the female hormones – oestrogen – may trigger an attack. This drop happens in the normal menstrual cycle, and because of this, after the change of life, women's migraine attacks tend to occur less often, once that their hormone levels are fairly constant.

One of the most common side-effects of the contraceptive pill is headache, and taking the Pill may make migraine worse, although a few women find that it helps. If your headaches get much worse and this coincides with your going on the Pill, you should discuss the matter with your family doctor, who may recommend an alternative contraceptive.

Your age The old belief that migraine tends to disappear as you grow older has some truth in it, but it is equally true to say that many people with migraine have it throughout their lives and that it may stay essentially the same.

However, it can change from the classical type to the common type or to a different variation of symptoms. In many patients, I have known it to disappear during their twenties, only to return in a different form later on in their lives.

How can you prevent an attack?

The first thing to do is to find out if there are any particular things which trigger an attack, and then avoid them if possible. Some of these may be obvious, but others can only be discovered if you keep a simple daily record of your activities over a period of a few attacks, noting such things as what you eat, what exercise you take, how much alcohol you drink and whether you watch television and how much.

Next you should try to ascertain how much warning of an attack you have. If the aura appears some hours before the actual headache, it is usually easy to start medication as soon as the warning starts, knowing that it will have time to be effective. If you only have a few minutes' warning, your medication can be given by injection and there is no reason why you should not do this yourself – thousands of diabetics give themselves injections every day of their lives. There are some medications that come as inhalers so that you can breathe them into your lungs in the same way as someone with asthma might; this is a very rapid method of preventing or relieving the symptoms.

There are other measures which can help. In particular, quiet and rest can be quite effective, and you should try to lie down in a darkened room if an attack is imminent. If your life-style is fairly stressful and migraine is becoming frequent or severe, you will have to think about what you can alter. It is not usually possible to give up a job which puts you under a lot of pressure but, if you can, it is certainly worth considering. Usually the best you can do is to identify the parts of your life-style which are stressful, and if you can change or eliminate them, you should do so. This may mean no more than taking life at a slightly more gentle pace whenever you can.

Drug treatment

For nausea If nausea and vomiting are what troubles you, there is one very good drug called metoclopramide which your doctor may well prescribe. It comes in pill form, or if the warning of the migraine attack is very short, it can be injected. It not only relieves the feeling of sickness but also helps the stomach to act normally so that any painkillers you might take afterwards will be absorbed more quickly. Two preparations are now available in Britain and Ireland which contain a combination of metoclopramide with a painkiller (Paramax and Migravess).

For pain The most common drugs used for this are aspirin and paracetamol (acetaminophen in the United States). Some people find that aspirin may upset their stomaches; if this happens, consult your doctor who may be able to prescribe an alternative.

For the attack The best drug to use initially is ergotamine tartrate (or dihydroergotamine), which helps to contract the affected blood vessels in the head and also acts against one of the body's chemicals which can trigger attacks. It is most effective when taken as soon as any symptoms arise, and can be inhaled or injected for fast relief.

Some of the pills containing ergotamine also contain other drugs which can be sedatives or anti-nausea drugs. Whatever type you take, you must understand that the ergotamine drugs are particularly powerful ones. In overdose, they produce very similar symptoms to migraine, such as headache, nausea and vomiting, and they can also affect your circulation, particularly in the tips of the fingers and toes. These are excellent drugs for migraine but you must be very careful with the dose you take. Some people who take too much ergotamine, think that the symptoms of overdose are merely their migraine: they are both the same.

For continuous preventive treatment If you have severe attacks of migraine or your job is threatened by too much sickness and being off work, you may be prescribed continuous medication. This will involve the regular taking of sedatives such as diazepam (Valium) in small doses and anti-migraine drugs like pizotifen (pizotyline in Canada), clonidine and methysergide. Although these anti-migraine drugs obtain their effects in different ways, they all act to stabilize the blood vessels. Your doctor may think it is worth trying them one by one until you find the best for you.

A word about methysergide: this is a powerful drug which in large quantities can cause fibrosis, or scarring, at the back of the chest, adversely affecting the blood flow in major arteries and veins. To avoid these side-effects, the dose should be kept as low as possible and taken for only about four months, with a break of at least one month. Methysergide is often the drug of last resort in migraine and often works well when nothing else has.

Acupuncture As the standard medications are normally effective for migraine, there is usually no point in using acupuncture – a technique of inserting fine needles into certain points in the skin to relieve pain. But it is worth trying if you have severe attacks or have long-term migraine, and other types of treatment have not worked.

The type of acupuncture we use for migraine at my pain-relief clinic involves only a few treatments to see if the patient is suitable for it and will benefit from it. If the patient has a headache when treated, we can tell if it will work after the first treatment. If not, we will probably have to wait until after the next expected attack. If the patient has been given some relief by the acupuncture, no more is given until the migraine returns or the headaches become severe again. Ideally, a patient should not need more than four treatments a year. I have found that about two-thirds of my patients with severe attacks or chronic migraine respond to acupuncture by having fewer and less severe attacks. (See pages 103–5 for more information on acupuncture.) For further details about migraine and other types of headache, consult *Migraine and Headaches* by Dr Marcia Wilkinson, another book in this series.

Other types of headache

Cluster headache
This condition, sometimes called migrainous neuralgia, is another type of headache due to unstable blood vessels. Migraine is sometimes called upper-half headache, while cluster headache is called lower-half headache. In other words, cluster headaches tend to affect your face while migraine has its effect higher up.

Cluster headache gets its name from its tendency to come in bouts or clusters. You have attacks every day for a few weeks which then die away for months at a time until another cluster of attacks occurs.

There are a number of differences between this type of headache and migraine. It is much less common than ordinary migraine – only about 5 per cent as many people suffer from it – and men are four times more likely to get it than women. The time during which the bouts last varies from a few weeks to a few months. The individual attacks usually start at the same time each day or, more commonly, night, and the clusters tend to occur seasonally, often in spring or autumn, disappearing during the rest of the year.

An attack can last up to two hours. Typically it takes about half an hour to reach its peak, lasts about one hour and then takes another half an hour to go. When the attack is at its peak, it is remarkably painful and can be anywhere in the head but is usually in the cheek or eye. The eye on the affected side becomes watery and red, while the nostril on that side often becomes blocked.

What can be done? The same anti-migraine drugs mentioned previously can be used for cluster headaches. As with migraine, it may be that ergotamine in pill form takes too long to be absorbed, so injecting the dose as soon as the attack starts is sometimes tried. As the attack often starts early in the morning, ergotamine suppositories (waxy cones containing the drug which are pushed into the back passage where they melt slowly, releasing the drug) inserted just before going to bed are very useful. As a last resort, methysergide is often found to be effective.

Tension headache
Anxiety or stress in one form or another can produce tension which, in turn, can produce a headache. A very ill child will often cause headaches in parents, and worry about work or losing your job is another common cause. People who are overmeticulous or those who are very conscientious about their homes, families or work may set themselves such high standards that these are impossible to attain, resulting in anxiety or stress or both, and this can produce a typical tension headache.

They are about 25 per cent as common as migraine.

Unlike migraine, the pain of a tension headache often lasts all day and gets worse throughout the day, and these headaches can develop only occasionally or may occur every day. The pain is often described as a weight pressing down on the head or as a tight band around the head. When severe, they tend to spread upwards from the forehead to the top of the head and may go all the way to the back of the neck. Sometimes they start in the forehead, then are also felt at the back of the head just above the neck, and as the day goes by, these two pains spread and ultimately join together. This happens because the scalp muscles form a continuous sheet from the forehead, over the top of the head and then to the back of the head. When you are tense, these muscles contract and stay contracted, especially if you are frowning with concentration. After a time, they have contracted for so long that they become painful. This is the reason why long-distance drivers tend to get tension headaches. They concentrate, holding their heads still for a long time, all the while being subjected to the stress of driving in busy traffic. The same features so obvious in the motorist cause most tension headaches, namely, the tightening of muscles and stress.

Drug treatment The first thing to do is to try to relieve the headache with simple painkillers, such as aspirin or paracetamol (acetaminophen in the US) in the recommended dose. But if the tension headache is severe and long-lasting, then no amount of pills is going to relieve the pain. That will only occur when you manage to free yourself of the tension. Yet there are many people who are taking two, three or more times the proper dose of painkillers because they think 'more is better' and will get rid of the pain. This is not so, but far more important is the fact that the long-term, continued use of drugs such as aspirin or paracetamol may produce, respectively, damage to the stomach lining and liver damage. Other problems can arise when such painkillers are mixed with each other or with other drugs (see Chapter 10). Therefore it is best to take reasonable doses (your doctor will tell you what these are) and not to mix the different types. It is believed that mixing different types of painkillers is especially bad for the kidneys.

Self-help So if pills do not relieve your tension headache, what will? Well, relaxation will usually do the trick. Most people suffering from such headaches are much better when they are on vacation, but unfortunately they cannot be on vacation all the year round, so you must find some other method or methods which you can use whenever you feel a tension headache coming on. For ideas on relaxation techniques, see pages 106–8.

Just being taught how to relax your muscles may be sufficient but, if not, biofeedback can be tried. You probably tend to perform better if you have something to measure your accomplishments against – for example, an athlete runs faster when there are other fast runners in a race – and this is the principle on which biofeedback works. You attach sensors to your fingers from a machine which measures your heart rate and how much you are sweating, among other things. As any of these increase, this shows on the machine either as an increasingly fast flashing light or a faster beeping noise. The object is to learn how to make the signal go slower, thus reducing the rate of some of your body functions. When you are tense, your heart beats faster and you sweat more (even though you may not be aware of it), and by con-

scious effort, it is possible to reduce these, thus lessening the tension you are feeling and the headache it is producing. Once you have mastered the technique, you will eventually be able to achieve the same results without the biofeedback machine.

Yoga, massage (see Chapter 12), hypnosis (see Chapter 11), meditation and other methods can all be used effectively to relieve stress and muscle tension, as most of them depend on relaxation of the body. Finally, as with migraine, you should try to remove stressful conditions from your life – often easier said than done.

Tense jaw headache
This pain occurs primarily because of tension, when you clench your teeth and continually tense the muscles which open and close the jaw, and it is a condition very similar to tension headache. In this condition, elaborately termed the masticatory dysfunction syndrome, 80 per cent of sufferers experience pain over one side of the face (in the remaining 20 per cent the pain is on both sides). The pain can spread from the temple over the angle of the jaw and involve the ear and the neck near that angle, but often the pain is in only part of this area. Usually the temperomandibular joint – where the jaw is hinged — is very painful to pressure.

People with this syndrome often clench their teeth during sleep and can then often be heard grinding them (this is technically called bruxism).

What can be done? Like tension headache, this pain can be relieved by any of the simple relaxation methods (see pages 106–8). If this is not enough, taking a tranquillizer such as diazepam (Valium) for a short period, combined with the wearing of an occlusal splint at night should be tried. The splint is a small, U-shaped, plastic appliance which fits over the biting surface of some of the teeth and prevents the jaws from coming together tightly. It is usually most effective in helping to relax the jaw muscles.

The same type of pain can be felt when your jaw overcloses because of loss of teeth and/or an alteration in the shape of your jaw, so that extra tension is put on the joint. The use of an occlusal splint and tranquillizers will also relieve this.

Hangover

'The morning after the night before' feeling is known to most of us, and if we have not experienced it ourselves, we are bound to know someone who has. Caused by taking too much alcohol into the body, in effect the hangover is produced by a slight case of alcohol poisoning.

By drinking too much in a short period of time, too much alcohol is absorbed into the bloodstream and overloads the body's 'depoisoning' ability. This is mostly carried out in the liver, so it is not surprising that we feel 'liverish' after a night out. Not only is the liver affected, but the stomach and the brain as well: the stomach from a direct assault on its lining and the brain from the effect of the alcohol on the nerve cells. In the brain, alcohol acts as an anaesthetic and that is why a drunk person is uncoordinated with slurred speech – he is half-anaesthetized.

In treating and trying to prevent the pain of a hangover, the following tips should be helpful:

Do
- Space out your drinking over a period of time.
- Drink soft drinks in between the alcoholic ones.
- Eat before drinking.
- Drink a pint (570 ml) or more of a sweet drink before going to bed – this will replace lost liquid and will help raise blood sugar levels.
- Take an antacid in the morning to settle your stomach.
- Take vitamin C (in pill or powder form, or in a fruit juice) which may help to break down the alcohol in your liver.
- Take a simple painkiller such as paracetamol (acetaminophen).

Don't
- Drink to excess if you can avoid it.
- Drink fizzy drinks or mixers as these tend to increase the rate at which alcohol is absorbed.
- Drink on an empty stomach.
- Mix your drinks.
- Take aspirin as this may further irritate your stomach lining.
- Drink alcohol to get rid of the hangover – the 'hair of the dog'. This only masks the symptoms and makes the final effects worse. It also encourages alcohol dependency.

Headaches caused by foods

There are many foods which can produce a headache in susceptible people. Ice cream and other cold foods can stimulate one of the nerves in the head, causing pain in the throat and the side of the head. Cured meats frequently contain chemicals called nitrites which can widen blood vessels and cause pain. Thus this type is sometimes called the 'hot-dog headache'. There is also one caused by an additive that many, particularly Chinese, restaurants use to increase the flavour of their food and which is present in soy sauce – monosodium glutamate. Often this headache is accompanied by nausea, abdominal pains and dizziness and this collection of symptoms has come to be known as 'Chinese restaurant syndrome'!

The best treatment for any of these is avoidance of the foods which cause them.

Eyesight and headaches

Poor vision does not of itself cause headache or eye-ache. If you have poor sight and screw up your eyes to see better while frowning and holding your head back and your neck stiff, it is no wonder that tension headache will result if you keep it up long enough. If light hurts your eyes, or they constantly tingle and smart, or one of them is painful, there is some other cause for this and you should visit your doctor.

Headaches caused by physical illness or injury

The body's functions are highly integrated, and when one part is hurt or diseased, this will often produce headache. All of the following circumstances in which headaches arise should be dealt with by the proper medical personnel.

Head injury Headaches commonly result from minor head injuries such as bumping your head against a kitchen cupboard, but these are usually mild and last only an hour or so. Oddly enough, severe headache does *not* usually occur in the serious head injuries caused by, say, traffic accidents. In fact, headaches occur in the victims of such accidents less often than in the population as a whole. As we have seen, pain is a subjective thing, and its presence in other injuries may make you oblivious to a relatively mild pain in the head. Headaches do occur as a result of the strain and anxiety placed on your life by an accident, but not usually from any physical damage.

Whiplash If you suffer a whiplash injury to the neck in a car accident, you may develop both neck-ache and headache. Often the headache is in the forehead, side of the head and around the eye, and the pain is a nagging ache which is made worse when the head or neck moves. See page 50 for treatment.

High blood pressure Very high blood pressure can cause a severe pounding headache which is worse in the morning but improves during the day when the head is raised and the blood pressure in it drops. Mild high blood pressure does not cause regular headaches, although one may occur if the pressure rises temporarily. Similarly, if your blood pressure falls due to relaxation and treatment, the headache also improves.

Brain tumour The possibility that their headaches are due to brain tumours worries most people. However, the symptoms of this are very different to those I have described previously, and they are also *very* rare, with less than 1 per cent of patients attending headache clinics being found to have such tumours – and such people only go to these clinics because they are not responding to treatment, and are thus a tiny minority of all people who have headaches.

A brain tumour may be suspected if a person has headaches that are worse in the morning and are aggravated by coughing, sneezing, bending down and exertion, especially if they are in someone over the age of fifty and the pain has been getting steadily worse over a relatively short time – say, three months or less. There may be vomiting and double vision as well, and sometimes drowsiness and weakness in a limb. As you can see, this set of symptoms is very different to anything described so far.

If you are worried about a headache which is getting steadily worse and which does not respond to treatment, do see your family doctor. Although this means that a lot of simple headaches will be investigated, it does ensure that the serious ones will not be missed. Your doctor or specialist will give you advice.

7. TOOTHACHE AND MOUTH PAIN

Toothache must be the most common severe pain which people encounter – especially in Western countries where consumption of sugar, which leads to tooth decay, is so high; although with the arrival of fluoride toothpastes and, in a few countries such as New Zealand, of fluoridation of the water supply, tooth decay and its accompanying problems are becoming less common than they once were. Recent research by Prof Ronald Melzack and others at McGill University in Canada rates the severity of toothache above the pain of arthritis (see diagram on page 19). This pain is also most successfully treated by the dental profession, as witness the fact that so few of us go about with dental pain, and if we do, it is rectified quickly and relatively easily. Because teeth are insensitive on the surface, it is easy to forget that they are living parts of the body, and pain in them can result from a number of different starting points.

The teeth
A tooth is made up of three layers (see diagram overleaf). The part that you can see is a very hard layer of enamel, which does not cover the whole of the tooth but stops a little way under the gum. Beneath the enamel and producing the shape of the tooth is a fairly hard substance called dentine, and in the centre of this is a soft fleshy region called the pulp. This last contains nerves and blood vessels and supplies chemicals and nutrients to the rest of the tooth material. There are connections between the dentine and the pulp

in the form of small tubes called dentinal tubules; the nutrients pass along these. The root of the tooth is set in the bone of the jaw, and the pulp receives nourishment through a small opening at each root's end. In children and young adults, these openings may be relatively large as the teeth are being replaced and growing to adult size.

How pain can arise

Heat and cold The first thing to understand is that pain can occur in the teeth without there being any damage or holes at all. Take, for instance, what happens when you eat something cold. Everybody knows that if you sink your front teeth into, say, ice cream, it is likely to hurt quite a bit. This is called thermal pain. This does not happen with everyone, but in some people the smaller teeth, such as the front teeth (the lower incisors) can become painful. This occurs when the nerves of the pulp are stimulated; and the area where this happens is believed to be where the dentine and pulp meet. If you take a small tooth and cover it with ice (or ice cream), after a short interval the cold will penetrate down to the dentine–pulp junction and you will feel pain. The same thing can sometimes happen with hot drinks.

In addition, the amount of enamel covering the teeth varies, with the enamel on the small front teeth being the thinnest, and these are usually the ones which feel thermal pain in this way. Some people also have less enamel than others, and this may be why they feel

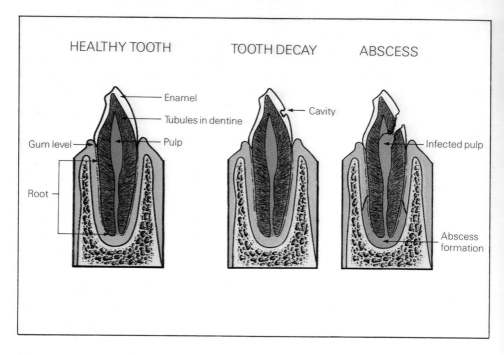

A normal tooth (left), a tooth with a cavity (centre), and an infected tooth with an abscess (right).

thermal pain more easily.

Tooth decay Naturally, if there is a break in the tooth surface – a hole caused by tooth decay (called caries) – or if the gum has receded exposing the dentine, the pain is felt more easily and quickly. Tooth decay is caused by acid formed by the action of bacteria on the sugar in food. This action takes place in the rough, sticky layer of plaque that coats your teeth. The acid destroys enamel and dentine, but contrary to what you might expect, the decay itself is not painful. Once the dentinal tubules are exposed by decay, thermal pain can occur as hot and cold drinks and food or cold air reach them. It takes a certain amount of time for the change in temperature to occur and also time for things to become normal again, and it is during this interval that sharp, throbbing pain is felt.

Fillings When areas of decay are found by dentists, they drill them away under a local anaesthetic (see Chapter 10) and then fill the resulting cavities with fillings. These have to withstand tremendous pressures during biting and so are usually made of metal. However, since this is a good conductor of heat and cold, dentists first have to put in a lining of cement which is a good insulator. If this were not done, you would feel pain every time you ate or drank.

The filling that is put in a tooth does not unite with the dentine but merely makes a very close contact with it. Unfortunately, the filling and the dentine expand slightly differently when they come in contact with heat, and contract slightly differently with cold. Thus a gap can develop between them, and this can vary quite appreciably since the temperature of food and drink can vary widely – from hot soup to ice cream. When a gap of this type exists, temperature changes have a much greater effect. And when substances with a high osmotic pressure – that is, those which have a tendency to draw in fluid – are eaten, such as a sugary substance like caramel, there is a high osmotic pressure in and around the gap and fluid is drawn through the dentinal tubules. The result is pain.

Finding the source of the pain One of the difficulties facing dentists when we arrive with toothache is that it is not always easy for them to know immediately which teeth are responsible. The problem of referred pain (see page 12) often complicates matters. Most of us know that when we have had a toothache for more than a few hours, the pain seems to spread all over one side of the face. It is impossible to point to the offending tooth in these circumstances, and all that we can do is to indicate the general area of pain.

X-rays may show the culprit by re-vealing an unexpected area of decay, but in a 'well-filled' mouth – and most of us have several previously filled teeth – it may be necessary to remove some of the old fillings before the cause of the pain can be revealed. It will probably turn out to be fresh decay developing underneath or by the side of an old filling.

Pain caused by infection
So far I have mostly talked about tooth pain produced by the effects of heat and cold. What about pain caused by infection? Acute inflammation results when dental decay reaches the pulp of a tooth. It can remain in one spot but usually spreads quickly throughout the whole pulp. As in any inflammation, there is then an increase in the blood flow as well as swelling from fluid passing out of the arteries and veins. The dental pulp is surrounded by tough, non-elastic dentine and enamel that cannot expand, and so the pressure in the tooth increases. Each time your heart beats, the pressure in the arteries

The most commonly used words from the McGill Questionnaire (page 18) to describe toothache.

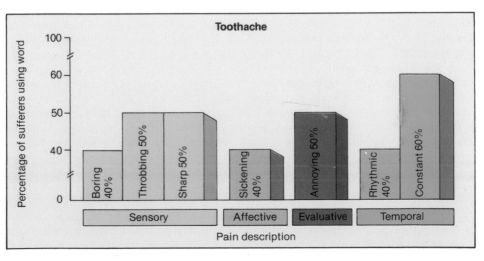

is raised for a moment and this increases the pressure in the pulp, and the pain that the infection has produced throbs in time to the heartbeat – a hallmark of this type of infection. This spreads and aches (with the throb on top) and can go on for hours. It is made worse by hot or cold drinks, by tapping the tooth or by pressure on the tooth when biting.

What can be done? A pulp infection is treated by removing that part of the pulp which is infected as early as possible. This procedure is called a pulpectomy. When the whole of the pulp is dead, either the tooth is removed (extracted) and this will allow the drainage of any infection, or just the pulp is removed through openings in the centre and tip of the tooth. These are repeatedly dressed and antibiotics are given until the infection subsides. When the infection has finally disappeared, the tooth is permanently filled. This process is very time-consuming and so is very expensive, but it does save the tooth.

What can happen if treatment is delayed? If inflammation of the pulp remains untreated, eventually the pulp dies and the pain disappears but, unfortunately, this usually means that the situation has become even more serious, as by that time the infection has passed through the end of the tooth into the surrounding bone. This is called a periapical infection. Periapical pain can also be present at the same time as the pain produced by an infected pulp, as these infections follow on from one another, or it can follow some time after the pulp has died and that pain has disappeared. Periapical pain is more common in children. The main difference between the two types of pain is that, in periapical pain, there is a continuous aching pain which is not made worse by hot or cold; like the pain of an infected pulp, it also throbs in time to the heartbeat, and biting on the tooth or tapping it makes it worse. The affected tooth is usually easily located by tapping it, but be careful if you try this as the pain it causes can be tremendous.

If this type of infection is not drained away, it will spread through the bone, and not only will you become ill from absorbing the poisons produced by the infection, but eventually the infection will find its own way out in the form of an abscess or gumboil (opposite).

Again the simplest method of controlling this type of infection is by extracting the tooth, and in severe cases this may have to be done. However, the affected tooth can usually be drained as I have already described.

First aid for toothaches
Because of the progressive damage that can be done by tooth decay and infection, it is vital that expert dental advice be sought as soon as you have any toothache. If you have to wait any time to see the dentist, the pain of a row of teeth can often be temporarily relieved by rinsing your mouth with a warm solution of bicarbonate of soda. Pain in one tooth can be eased by filling any hole created by decay with a piece of cotton wool dipped in oil of cloves or a similar preparation. Your pharmacist should be able to give you good advice on what to use.

Tips on preventing toothache
Of course, the best way to avoid toothache is to brush your teeth regularly and eat a proper diet, so that you have healthy teeth with a minimal amount of decay or other problems. The following guidelines should help to cut down your visits to the dentist's chair:
- Brush your teeth at least twice a day – after breakfast and before bedtime, and preferably after every meal.

- Make sure your toothbrush is small enough to get into all the crevices, and is in good enough condition to remove the plaque thoroughly from your teeth's surfaces.
- Use a fluoride toothpaste to harden the enamel and reduce decay.
- Brush up and down, and from side to side, and don't forget to brush the gums too.
- Use dental floss – tough thread that is often waxed – after meals to remove plaque and food from between your teeth.
- Try to eliminate, or at least greatly cut down on sugary foods and drinks in your diet. If you do eat something sweet, brush your teeth as soon as possible afterwards.
- Have a dental check-up every six months. That way, your dentist has a good chance of dealing with decay before it gets to the painful stage. He or she will also be able to give you regular preventive treatment, such as descaling and polishing.

Gumboils and abscesses

A gumboil is the final stage of a tooth infection, and usually takes the form of an abscess (a swelling that is filled with infected fluid) between the inside of the cheek and the gum. Everyone who does not go for regular dental treatment is likely to have at least one abscess at some time in their lives. Any form of treatment to relieve the gumboil's pain and inflammation is really only a stop-gap measure, and the removal of the infection's cause – the tooth or just the infected pulp – as outlined above is the only really effective treatment.

Children may also develop gumboils but these seem to be less painful, as their teeth do not extend as deeply into the gums and bone as in adults, and the roots of their first set of teeth are being absorbed before they get their second set. Therefore, any infection is nearer the surface and drainage is easier. Dentists usually wait before treating these until they can do a number of items of dental hygiene at the same time, so that the child only has to have one anaesthetic for all the treatment. Having to wait to have their gumboils treated does not seem to upset children.

Dry socket

Although uncommon, this can be a most painful condition which occurs after a tooth has been extracted. After extraction, the socket normally fills up with blood which then clots and gradually changes to form bone. Sometimes the clot may not form properly or may break up too soon – for example, because of too vigorous mouth washing. In these cases, a dry or empty socket results, and a spreading, intense, dull-aching type of pain develops in the region of the extraction within forty-eight hours.

The treatment is to wash away the food debris which has inevitably accumulated in the socket, and then the socket is packed with gauze and a paste. This pack allows the socket to heal gradually from the bottom up and the pain disappears very rapidly.

Teething

Babies First teeth usually emerge at about six months or so, and the baby may begin to suffer some mild discomfort as each new one cuts through. Sometimes he or she will develop a small red patch on the cheek over the tooth or a slightly red gum, but often nothing is apparent except that the infant is restless and weepy.

The lucky majority of babies seem to suffer little or no pain, but the rest must endure it until around the age of two and a half, when most or all of their first set of teeth have come through.

Parents should try to comfort and distract their teething babies, and perhaps give them children's paracetamol (acetaminophen in the United States) as a painkiller at night if the discomfort prevents them from sleeping or wakes them up. Biting on something hard is also helpful, and you can give your baby a hard or water-filled teething ring, carrot or rusk. There are some proprietary teething creams and gels containing small doses of local anaesthetic which seem to have some effect, but this is fairly short-lived as babies tend to dilute the preparations as they salivate and drool.

Never give a teething baby anything sugary to suck as this will harm his or her growing teeth, and *always* consult your doctor if your baby develops fever or diarrhoea or loses his appetite, as these are almost never caused by teething.

Teenagers and adults Most people think of teething as a problem that only affects babies. But the teething pain in the back upper and lower jaw caused by a wisdom tooth coming through the gums can be experienced by anyone over the age of fourteen. Wisdom teeth have usually appeared by the age of twenty-four, although they are sometimes cut even later.

The pain gradually builds up to an intense level, and usually lasts for between a week and ten days, until the tooth cuts through the surface of the gum, at which point the pain fades away. Simple painkillers like aspirin and paracetamol should relieve the discomfort, and biting on something hard will help to reduce the pain.

Mouth ulcers
Apart from the small ulcers which can occur when you bite the inside of your cheek or when a rough denture rubs against it and which heal quickly and are relatively painless, some people get what are called aphthous ulcers. They occur frequently in adolescents and young adults, and affect more women than men. The ulcers are usually small (about 2 mm square) and white, although they sometimes look yellow on a red base, and they cause mild pain which increases with eating – especially with acidic or spicy food. They appear a few at a time and heal within a few days.

Their cause is unknown so the only way to deal with them is to treat the symptoms they cause. There are various substances which your doctor may prescribe to put on ulcers as a protective covering, such as carboxymethyl cellulose, and sometimes a steroid drug is added which acts to reduce the inflammation. A choline salicylate paste can also be used, or small pills of hydrocortisone hemisuccinate can be dissolved in the mouth to reduce the inflammation. Gargling with a weak saline solution may also soothe the discomfort.

Cold sores
One of the two main types of herpes virus – herpes simplex – causes blisters to form around the mouth which are popularly called cold sores. First there are small swellings full of fluid which then burst and form scabs. Before the scabs are complete, they form ulcers which are painful but eventually heal completely. Once the herpes virus has infected the skin, it lies dormant until it is triggered by something such as a cold, the flu, a sore throat or even sunlight, when the virus becomes reactivated and another crop of cold sores results. There is no cure for these, and the only treatment is to let them run their course, although your doctor may prescribe a preparation such as idoxuridine that may relieve the itchiness and pain.

8. WOMEN AND PAIN

There are two acute pains to which women as a group are usually prone. One is the pain of childbirth, and the other is menstrual or period pain – dysmenorrhoea.

Period pain

This usually occurs at the beginning or just before menstruation and continues until menstruation is well advanced. Probably 50 per cent of all women suffer from period pain at some stage in their lives, and in approximately 9 per cent of them it is sufficiently severe for them to need a day or two off school or work. Dysmenorrhoea usually develops shortly after a girl begins to menstruate and tends to taper off after the age of twenty-five. It used to be said that childbirth solves this problem; it may do so in many cases but certainly not in all, and a few women go through life with this difficulty.

The pain is caused by strong contractions of the muscular uterus wall. A number of natural chemicals are released within the uterus before and during menstruation, and it is believed that some women produce a kind of prostaglandin (see page 9) which makes the muscles of the uterus contract painfully. Other theories are that some of these women do not produce enough of the hormone progesterone, or that they are not taking in enough vitamin B₆ (pyridoxine).

Although most women experiencing period pain tend to have it disappear in their twenties, there is a second kind which can suddenly start in women over thirty. It is often associated with other pelvic problems such as infection, fibroids and so on, and because of this, it should always be investigated by a doctor.

Treatment The simplest method of dealing with period pain is to take a painkiller such as paracetamol (acetaminophen in the United States) or aspirin; the latter has the added benefit of acting against prostaglandins. A combined pill of paracetamol and codeine is quite powerful (there are several over-the-counter preparations available) and it is often worth while trying one to start with and, if that is not effective, taking a second after forty-five minutes. Two pills make some women feel a little dopey. If you have severe pain, you may have to rest and take more powerful painkillers prescribed by your doctor (see Chapter 10).

Those women who have taken aspirin for its anti-prostaglandin effect but for whom it has not worked may find that they respond better to other anti-prostaglandin drugs such as mefenamic acid (which seems to be particularly effective in period pain), ibuprofen or indomethacin – drugs that are also used to counter the inflammation of arthritis.

Other types of drug treatment which have had some effect in some women are the taking of the hormone progesterone (or its synthetic counterpart, progestogen) to correct any imbalance in the hormone level; and the taking of vitamin B_6 (pyridoxine) which has the advantage of being available over the counter. The latter is also used to treat the symptoms of pre-menstrual syndrome (PMS). And, of course, if you take the contraceptive pill, you generally avoid painful periods by stopping the process by which prostaglandins are released: you do not ovulate and you have only 'artificial' periods.

Other methods that have been successfully used by some women to overcome painful periods are electrical stimulation, heat treatment, exercise and relaxation techniques (see Chapters 11 and 12).

Another important aspect to keep in mind is that Western culture has, over the centuries, considered menstruation to be 'unclean' and 'the curse', and any embarrassment or shame that you may feel about it may, in fact, increase the amount of pain you experience. By learning as much about your body as possible and by coming to realize that periods are as natural as, say, growing your first tooth, you may find that you will feel less pain.

Childbirth

There are a number of mistaken ideas about the pain of childbirth which it is important to dispel. The most important of these is the idea that, although childbirth is usually painful, if a woman does her antenatal exercises and learns to do a relaxation method properly, all will be well and she will feel little or no pain. This is simply not so. Also, it is often argued that as the uterus normally contracts, its action in childbirth is quite normal and therefore should not be painful. Well, it is painful. If, say, your bowels, which normally contract to pass food along, become constipated and start working against a resistance, you soon feel pain.

There are some women, it is true, (between 7 and 14 per cent) who do not feel much or any pain during childbirth. They are the lucky ones. They do not need natural childbirth techniques or anything else to help them. But for the majority, the pain of childbirth is very severe – one of the worst pains that human beings ever have to put up with. Probably the most graphic description of it is that it is like the pain of trying to pass a melon through the bowel! The strange thing is that women themselves tend not to talk about the severity of this pain. This is partly because the human mind forgets what it does not want to remember, and is also due to the fact that, because most babies are wanted, the pleasure in the new baby tends to swallow up the pain.

Pain in childbirth arises from two areas. One is the body of the uterus in which the child lies, and the other is the lower part of the uterus (the cervix), the vagina and the surrounding muscles and tissues which together form the birth canal. The process of childbirth involves the uterus contracting rhythmically. These contractions pull on the cervix until it begins to open up and then the baby and its surrounding amniotic sac filled with fluid are gradually pushed through it. The nerves to the uterus come from the middle of the spinal cord so the sharp, cramping pain of the contractions is felt relatively high up in the back in the upper part of the lumbar region (around the back of the waist).

Once the cervix has expanded enough for the child's head (the largest part of the baby) to come through, the baby starts to push its way to the outside by stretching the birth canal in its path. Naturally, this cannot be anything but painful. But, after the birth canal has been stretched once, it is easier for it to stretch again, and this is why women having another child have

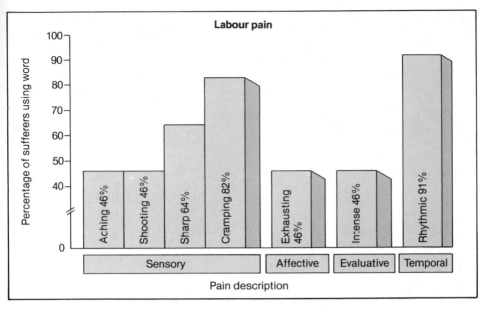

The most commonly used words from the McGill Questionnaire (page 18) to describe labour pain.

an easier time on the second and subsequent occasions.

Prof Ronald Melzack has used his McGill Pain Questionnaire (see pages 18–19) to determine the amount of pain felt by women in childbirth. He had found that the levels of the 'pain rating index' (PRI) – the total made up of the values given to the descriptive words the sufferers chose – for some common types of pain were: back pain and cancer about 28, and toothache and arthritis around 20. Asking women to fill in the pain questionnaire in between contractions – while the women were in the process of labour – the PRI score for women having first babies was around 34 and for those having second and subsequent babies was 30. All the women did not fall into this range, some extending above and below it. In first-time mothers, about 65 per cent of the women had pain scores of between 22 and 41, about 10 per cent had pain below a score of 21 and about 25

per cent were above 42. This is a very high level of pain indeed.

Because of the universality of this severe pain, doctors and others have devoted themselves to trying to discover ways of alleviating or eliminating it.

Antenatal training

Antenatal ('before birth') classes aim to do two things: to reduce the fear of labour by explaining to you how your body is changing and what to expect when you are in labour; and to teach two types of body control – exercises to help control breathing and those which are thought to improve muscle control and relaxation. These methods comprise what is called psychoprophylaxis (controlling pain using the mind), or natural childbirth, and they aim to reduce or eliminate the use of drugs and other 'artificial' pain relief, such as acupuncture and electrical nerve stimulation (see Chapter 11), during labour.

How effective is it? Performing these exercises while giving birth acts as a distraction to the pain and relaxes you so you do not experience the pain quite so acutely. Many women find them to be relatively effective.

The question of what effect antenatal training has had on labour pain was considered in Prof Melzack's study. He found that, while there is no doubt that this training makes a difference which can be measured by the questionnaire and which is statistically significant, it does not reduce the pain to very low levels. Prof Melzack's work showed that twenty-six first-time mothers with *no* antenatal training suffered pain with an average score of 37, while sixty-one women *with* childbirth training experienced pain with a score of about 33. This lower rate is still a higher score than that experienced by those suffering from the pain of cancer.

The fact that women still feel pain even though they conscientiously train for childbirth can have a number of consequences. Because many women expect too much of antenatal training, they can feel very let down when they find that childbirth is extremely painful despite all their efforts. They may panic, wondering what is going wrong. They may also feel that they are letting down all the people who have spent so much time in training them, and they may even wonder what is wrong in themselves.

Much, though, depends on the woman herself and those medical personnel helping her. If she has not got a low level of pain tolerance, feels prepared for what is to come and is treated as an intelligent, participating adult by doctors and midwives, she may feel the pain a great deal but may be able to handle it better. Antenatal training is important and beneficial, but don't feel guilty if you ask for pain relief during labour, even if you had planned not to. Among the group of mothers studied by Prof Melzack, over 80 per cent of those who had received antenatal training were given epidural anaesthesia.

Pain relief during labour

Between 50 and 60 per cent of women are given some sort of painkiller during childbirth, either by choice or sometimes, unfortunately, without any choice; the remaining 30 to 40 per cent may try another method. Although all the following drugs cross the placenta and pass to the baby, when they are given at suitable times in correct doses, the effects on the baby are minimal and short-lived.

Tranquillizers such as promazine and diazepam (Valium) may be given if a woman has high blood pressure or is particularly anxious. They should be avoided if possible.

Pethidine (meperidine in the United States) may be given when contractions are well advanced and painful. It is injected into a muscle and reduces the pain within twenty minutes, lasting from two to five hours.

Gas in the form of 'gas-and-air' (nitrous oxide – 'laughing gas' – and oxygen) or Trilene is usually offered at the end of the first stage of labour and at the beginning of the second (when the baby descends the birth canal and is born). It is taken in light doses via a face mask, and it has the advantage of being used by the woman herself, to control her own pain.

A pudendal block is a series of injections of a local anaesthetic given right before delivery. They are made just inside the vagina in the pudendal nerve, numbing the lower third of the birth canal and the external genitals.

Epidural anaesthesia In this, an anaesthetic is injected into the epidural space between the spinal cord and the vertebrae which surround it. When a thin tube (catheter) is placed there, the anaesthetic can be topped up as necessary. This method results in almost painless childbirth, with the woman numb from the waist down, but otherwise fully conscious. However, it must be performed only by a specially trained anaesthetist (anaesthesiologist in the United States). The drug may cause vomiting or a drop in blood pressure, and sometimes, because a woman feels no pain, she may be less able to push during the final stages and thus labour may take longer and forceps deliveries are more common.

Another recent development is the use of epidural anaesthesia during Caesarean section deliveries (see below) so that you can still be fully awake.

Over the years doctors have spent a great deal of time successfully developing methods of relieving pain in childbirth, from the first nitrous oxide 'gas–air' machine to the modern technique of local epidural anaesthesia. These methods carry small risks, so it is quite important that women should try to have their babies completely naturally, provided that the risks of so doing do not outweigh the risks of pain relief. It seems to me that, before women go into labour, they should be given more truthful information about what they can expect and should be taught to accept the help that is available if the pain of labour becomes unbearable.

Pain after childbirth

After the birth of your child, you will naturally be tired. It may be painful to urinate for the first twenty-four hours or so and the whole area between your legs may be sore. After delivery, the uterus often continues to contract, primarily to deliver the afterbirth, but sometimes these after-pains continue for the first few days, particularly in women who have had more than one child. They may be strongest during breastfeeding and are a good sign that the uterus is reducing to its former size. Painkillers such as aspirin will usually provide enough relief, without having any adverse effect on the baby via the breast milk.

Episiotomies This is a surgical incision, carried out as the baby's head appears, to cut the perineum (the skin between the vagina and anus). This is performed to avoid a jagged tear which, rarely, may extend into the anus itself, and is stitched up afterwards. After the birth, many women find that their episiotomies cause some or a lot of pain. In a recent study of 1,800 women carried out in Britain by the National Childbirth Trust, 65 per cent had had episiotomies. Many of them complained of pain during the stitching and of pain of varying severity for days afterwards, making it difficult to sit. About 20 per cent complained of pain on sexual intercourse for at least three months.

To help the cut heal and to relieve the pain, take hot salt baths. Pelvic floor exercises, which you may been taught at antenatal classes and involve tightening the muscles in that area as if stopping urinating in mid-stream, will aid healing too. Try also to eat high-fibre foods, such as unrefined bread and cereals, vegetables and fruit, to help make passing motions as pain-free as possible. It may be reassuring for you to look at your stitches with the aid of a mirror, to see that the incision is healing and that it was really only a small one.

Caesarean section After a Caesarean delivery, there is pain from the incision, and postnatal after-pains may feel worse because your abdomen is already sore. In some hospitals, if you have been under epidural anaesthesia during

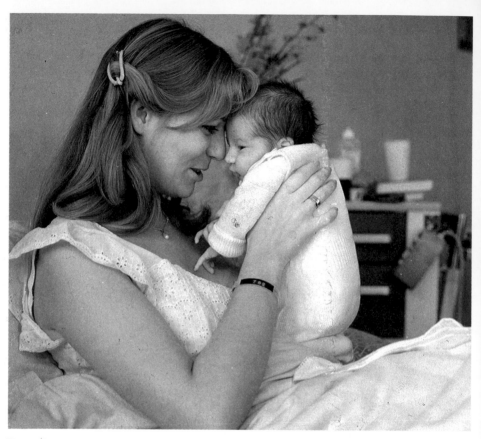

The pains of labour are soon forgotten once you start to enjoy your new baby.

the birth, the tube, or catheter, may be left in position in your spine so that the anaesthetic can be topped up to carry you through the first, most painful hours in the postnatal ward. Once the epidural catheter is removed and the anaesthetic has worn off you should be given painkillers – strong ones at first, such as pethidine (see page 93), then milder ones, such as aspirin or paracetamol (acetaminophen in the United States) – to relieve the soreness. Although a certain amount of these drugs will pass to the baby in the breast milk, they won't harm him in any way.

Apart from the pain of the incision, you may also experience discomfort from the bladder. During the operation, a catheter will have been placed in your bladder, and even when this has been removed you may feel cramp when your bladder is full.

To avoid painful straining when you go to the lavatory, try to eat as much high-fibre food as you can after the birth. To increase the roughage content of hospital food, it is a good idea to have your own supply of bran. Without a high-fibre diet you may need to take a laxative.

Sneezing, coughing or laughing will be painful for a time, but will not open your incision. It helps if you gently support your scar with both hands. Throughout your stay in hospital relaxation will help to prevent your body tensing up and increasing the pain (see Chapter 12 for relaxation techniques).

9. OTHER TYPES OF PAIN

It is clearly not possible in a book of this size to look closely at every variety of pain suffered by the human race, as that task would require several volumes. Throughout, I have concentrated on the commonest painful conditions, and those over which sufferers can take most positive and active control. Before moving on to describe the professional and self-help methods of pain relief that benefit nearly all types of pain in Chapters 10, 11 and 12, I want first to examine several more conditions, which although they do not each need a chapter to themselves, nevertheless cause pain to millions of people every year. Fortunately, in nearly all, the pain can either be got rid of altogether, or at least reduced to a tolerable level.

Facial nerve pain
The medical term for this is trigeminal neuralgia. A neuralgia is a pain along a nerve, and this type – also called *tic douleurex* – runs along a branch of the trigeminal nerve on one side of the face, affecting the forehead, cheek, lips and jaw. The pain flickers in the face like lightning. It can be the most severe of pains, usually intensely sharp, cutting or burning in character. It lasts about a minute and can be triggered by moving the jaw during eating or talking, washing the face or even just by a cold draught, and thus prevents you from eating, talking or washing. Afterwards, the skin over the painful area may be swollen and feels tender and stiff. Facial neuralgia is more common in women than in men and in those over the age of fifty. It is one of the few pains that is so intense that the sufferer may try to commit suicide if it is not treated.

In the past, this neuralgia was treated by permanently numbing the nerve via an injection of alcohol or by surgically cutting it but, unfortunately, about 10 per cent of those treated in this way developed another pain in the numb part of the face. More successful has been the recent use of either the drug carbamazepine (which seems to hinder the sudden discharge of nerve pain activity) or the technique of only partially destroying the nerve, leaving some sensation behind.

Abdominal pain
Pain in the abdominal area – anywhere between the bottom of the rib cage and the groin – can be caused by many different conditions, and it usually takes a doctor to sort out one from another. Here are some of the most common:

Hiatus hernia This occurs when the lower end of the oesophagus – the gullet – or the upper part of the stomach protrudes through a thin sheet of muscle called the diaphragm, which separates the abdomen from the chest. This happens because the muscles of the oesophagus at this juncture have become weakened.

Hiatus hernia may give little if any trouble, perhaps causing only indigestion and hiccups. But usually it produces painful heartburn, which is inflammation of the oesophagus, known by doctors as oesophagitis. The pain is caused by acid coming up from the stomach, resulting in a burning feeling behind the breastbone (sternum), which gets worse when you bend down or lie flat. This condition is quite common, and occurs more often in women, especially during pregnancy, and in the middle-aged, particularly if you are overweight.

Losing weight is the most effective thing you can do. Meanwhile, taking over-the-counter antacids will help to relieve the heartburn, as will avoiding bending, using several pillows at night (or raising the head of your bed a few inches off the ground), and not drinking just before bedtime.

If the problem persists, your doctor can prescribe other drugs which reduce the level of acid in your stomach. As a last resort you may be advised to have an operation to repair the hernia. You can be out of hospital within two to five days, and back at work in a few weeks. To help prevent recurrence, you should not lift heavy weights for at least twelve weeks after the operation, and should not be overweight.

Gastritis This is the medical term for inflammation of the stomach. It is usually caused by eating highly spiced foods or drinking an excess of alcohol, both of which can irritate the lining of the stomach, producing an indigestion-like pain and sickness. Smoking can also sometimes be implicated and certain drugs such as aspirin are known to be irritating (see Chapter 10). Just about everyone has an attack of gastritis at some time in their lives. You usually lose your appetite, become nauseated and vomit and there may be heartburn (see above). A mainly fluid, light diet for a few days usually allows the stomach to rest and apart from

avoiding the cause of the attack, this is normally all that is needed.

If the cause of the trouble is bacterial food poisoning, an allergy, or a virus, the disease is called gastroenteritis. The symptoms, which usually last for about two days, include those for gastritis plus diarrhoea and an intermittent severe cramping pain in the abdomen. In general, the symptoms are treated rather than the disease, and the main concern is the replacement of lost fluid, by giving plenty of water or fruit juice to drink, especially in infants and young children. Bad diarrhoea can be treated with kaolin, which solidifies the faeces, and painful spasm of the muscles of the intestines can be relieved by drugs which work on the nerves supplying these muscles. The widely used kaolin-and-morphine combination performs both these tasks. After a day or two without food, a bland diet should be eaten. You should avoid taking painkillers or antibiotics for both plain gastritis and gastroenteritis as these drugs only aggravate the condition.

Gallstones The gallbladder is located just below the liver and is connected to the common bile duct through which the bile produced by the liver passes on its way to the duodenum (the first part of the intestines). Some of this bile is stored in the gallbladder and there it may form into gallstones. About 10 per cent of people over the age of fifty develop these, and they are more common in fair, overweight women over forty.

Around a half of gallstones do not produce pain and are symptomless. But if a stone blocks the common bile duct this will cause very severe pain in the upper right-hand side of the abdomen (biliary colic), which builds up over several hours and then dies away. There will also be a high fever and sweating. The bile that cannot get through to the duodenum enters the bloodstream and your skin becomes yellowish (jaundiced) and the urine turns dark brown or orange. Rarely a gallbladder can become inflamed, often as a complication of stones. This is called cholecystitis and affects only around 0.1 per cent of the population each year. In acute cases, there is severe pain in the right side of the abdomen just under the rib cage, going backwards under the shoulder-blade, often with fever and vomiting.

These are two of the few abdominal complaints for which you can take painkillers without aggravating the condition. If you have biliary colic, you may be advised to have an operation in which the gallbladder is removed and the bile duct is cleaned surgically. The gallbladder, like the spleen and appendix (see overleaf), can be removed without making a difference to your well-being. You will probably be in hospital for about two weeks and should be able to resume normal activities within a couple of months.

An attack of cholecystitis is usually settled by a course of antibiotics. Sometimes drugs can be used to try to dissolve the stone(s) but in most cases surgical removal of the gallbladder is the only permanent solution.

Peptic ulcers These are gaps in the lining of the stomach or the duodenum (the first section of the small intestine) which cause pain ranging from a slight hunger-type pang to a piercing knife-like pain. It can be felt in a specific place – usually just under the breast bone (sternum) – but usually it is more vague, covering the upper abdomen, the lower chest or elsewhere. Gastric, or stomach, ulcer pains are usually made worse by eating, while duodenal ulcer pain may be relieved by food. Nausea, vomiting, loss of appetite and heartburn (oesophagitis) are other common symptoms. More than one in

A gallstone blocking the common bile duct produces a severe, knife-like pain which spreads backwards through the body to below the shoulder blade.

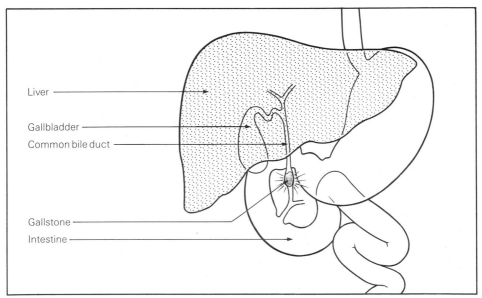

Liver

Gallbladder

Common bile duct

Gallstone

Intestine

ten of the Western population will develop a peptic ulcer at some time in their lives. The condition is very much more common in men than women, and mostly affects young and middle-aged adults.

Peptic ulcers tend to come and go naturally, and their recurrence may coincide with stress. Treatment is usually with acid-lowering drugs and antacids as well as those which cover the lining of the stomach and duodenum and aid healing. It is now known that diet has little or nothing to do with either causing ulcers or aiding in their healing, but a regular, balanced diet is to be recommended. Smoking and drinking alcohol – both of which can worsen an already existing ulcer – should be cut out completely, and most painkillers, particularly aspirin, and other anti-inflammatory drugs, such as steroids and those used to treat arthritis, should be avoided. If ulcers recur or if there are complications such as excessive bleeding, surgery may very rarely be necessary, but this has become much less common now that more effective drugs are available.

Appendicitis The appendix is a small redundant tube of gut at the junction between the small and large intestines. If it becomes inflamed by infection from bacteria, it results in the condition called appendicitis. This is rare in those under the age of two and over the age of thirty, and is most common in teenagers. Around one Western person in five hundred has appendicitis in any one year. It may be caused by the lack of fibre ('roughage') in the diet which slows down digestion and which, in turn, can lead to blockages in the appendix. In areas in which high-fibre diets are eaten such as Asia, Africa and Polynesia, the condition is relatively unknown, whereas in Western countries with refined diets, it is becoming increasingly common.

In the early stages, the pain of acute appendicitis is difficult to distinguish from plain stomach ache. There are colicky pains around the navel that come and go as the appendix contracts trying to remove any obstruction. After about six to twelve hours, the inflammation becomes more advanced and the lining of the abdomen (the peritoneum) becomes irritated. Sharp pain is then felt in the lower right abdomen. However, the location of the pain can vary, so any severe pain in the abdomen should be investigated by a doctor. Constipation, nausea and vomiting are common symptoms, and you may be in pain if you stretch your right leg down from the hip, as the appendix sometimes lies on the leg muscle where it joins the back.

Recurrent bouts of less severe appendicitis produce a 'grumbling' appendix. The part of the intestines near the appendix may surround it to wall off the infection, and this may become stuck to the appendix after the attack, infection flaring up from time to time.

No home treatments such as painkillers or laxatives should be tried and you should see a doctor as soon as possible. If he or she is reasonably sure that the cause of the pain and other symptoms is acute appendicitis, your appendix will have to be removed at once. If it is not removed, it may burst and all the infected material inside it will infect the abdominal lining, causing peritonitis. This is very dangerous, particularly in children under ten. You will probably have to stay in hospital for five to ten days, and you will be able to resume a normal life about a month after the operation.

If 'grumbling' appendix is diagnosed, the decision to have an operation may well be left with you. I would say that unless the pain is at an unacceptable level, it is not worth undergoing surgery that is not absolutely essential. Try to live with the pain – using some of the pain relief techniques in Chapters 11 and 12 – if it is not adversely affecting your health.

Shingles and afterwards

Shingles is caused by the same virus as chickenpox – herpes zoster – but shingles is a disease of adults, and the older you are, the more likely you are to get it. Between the ages of fifty and sixty, about five people per thousand contract it and this rate doubles after the age of eighty. Most of those who get shingles have had chickenpox. The virus lies dormant in the nerves – especially in those which run from the spinal cord around the chest and in those which supply the face – until it flares up when over the years resistance to it has fallen.

At first, you feel generally unwell and have tenderness on the skin over the affected nerves, usually around one-half of the body like a belt (the Greek *herpes zoster* means 'creeping girdle'). The sharp, burning pain in the skin gets worse and the skin reddens over a few days, then a rash breaks out which develops into liquid-filled blisters that half-encircle the body, commonly from the breast bone to the spine. The pain can be very severe, and is especially bad in the elderly. After a week or two, the blisters dry up and form scabs which drop off. The rash, blisters and pain can also occur on the face, particularly around the eye, but the eye itself and the ear can also be affected.

There is no really effective treatment for shingles and neither can it be prevented. Painkillers are usually given and the affected area is treated with idoxuridine – an antiviral liquid – at as early a stage as possible. In 70 per cent of people with shingles painting idoxuridine on to the blisters shortens the course of the disease. They quickly dry into scabs and the pain subsides.

In some unfortunate cases, the pain in the nerves continues even after the rash has disappeared, the herpes zoster virus having not only infected the nerves but destroyed some of the large A-beta nerve fibres (see page 11), which carry most tactile sensations. Once these A-beta fibres are destroyed, only the thin A-delta and C fibres remain, which carry only pain. And so every sensation from the area of the body with damaged large A-beta fibres will be a painful sensation. Even the feeling of clothes on the skin will be painful. This is post-herpetic neuralgia. Most people who get shingles do not get this, but there is no doubt that the older you are, the more chance there is of this complication. In fact, in those people over eighty years old who get shingles, more than half get post-herpetic neuralgia. The pain usually dies down after six months or so, but in those who get it severely, it can continue for the rest of their lives.

Anti-viral treatment The immediate treatment is to paint an anti-viral substance such as idoxuridine on to the affected area. This is believed to be absorbed into the nerves and thus to protect them from further damage by the virus. This treatment works for three out of every four sufferers.

Sympathetic nerve block In those who are particularly at risk – that is, the elderly – a sympathetic nerve block can be performed. Preliminary studies show that this stops the immediate pain of shingles in about two-thirds of patients, and if it returns, the procedure can be repeated. This treatment is believed to prevent the development of post-herpetic neuralgia.

The sympathetic nerves release a chemical in the body called noradrenaline (norepinephrine in the United States) which stimulates the nerve fibres and causes pain. It is not necessary to destroy permanently the sympathetic nerves to treat post-herpetic neuralgia at the early shingles stage. Temporary blocking can be carried out with simple local anaesthetics.

As this method may prevent the development of post-herpetic pain, and as it may relieve the acute stage of shingles as well, there is a lot to be said for carrying it out on all patients. But not every doctor is used to performing sympathetic blocks so these are not universally available, although most anaesthesiologists will be familiar with them, especially if they are associated with a pain relief clinic.

Epidural injection Another type of injection used for relieving the pain of shingles and also given to prevent the development of post-herpetic neuralgia is the epidural injection. I have already described how a local anaesthetic injected into the epidural space around the spinal cord produces the epidural block which is so useful in childbirth (see page 82). But for shingles, an anti-inflammatory steroid drug is injected, and in an unknown way, this may prevent the development of post-herpetic neuralgia. Again, there is no guarantee of this, but it does work in a reasonable percentage of patients. It may be that when the steroid drug is placed so close to the nerves entering the spinal cord, it manages to damp down the infection which can damage them and lead to long-term pain.

Steroids which help can also be given by mouth or by injection. They can certainly relieve the condition and prevent the post-herpetic pain in many cases, but because they affect your immune system, this can result in the infection spreading, so doctors use them very carefully.

Other drugs include a narcotic called buprenorphine (Temgesic in Britain), which is said to be less addictive (see page 93), and the newer antibiotics, such as acyclovir, which can destroy viruses and are used in virus infections. These are very powerful substances and are not without risk.

Cancer pain

Cancerous cells are not recognized as invaders by the body so the normal reaction of inflammation and pain does not occur when they are present. It is only when a tumour gets very large that it presses on a part of the body and then causes pain, and this is almost always in the later stages of the disease.

As we have seen, mood can severely affect the amount of pain you feel and vice versa. People with cancer understandably become very depressed and miserable. In the worst cases, with pain confining them to bed, they withdraw into themselves and cannot be bothered to take an interest in themselves, their personal appearance or any of the things which, before their illness, they were happy to do. This continues until their pain is relieved and it is surprising how quickly they can revert to their normal behaviour once that happens.

What can be done? Of all the severe chronic pains, the pain of cancer is the one most easily treated. Methods which involve preventing one or other of the pain pathways from working (either the pain-carrying nerves in the spinal cord or the small C fibres), in order to prevent pain transmission, are ideally useful in treating cancer pain. This does not mean that all cancer pain can be treated successfully, but if one type of treatment does not work, there is usually another which can be tried. Even if the pain cannot be relieved entirely, it can often be reduced considerably so that less powerful pain-relieving drugs can be used. There is great advantage in doing this, as the less powerful a drug is, the less chance there is of unpleasant side-effects. In the next chapter I shall be looking at pain-relieving drugs in detail.

10. PAIN-RELIEVING DRUGS AND ANAESTHETICS

Drugs

For most people in pain, drugs are the first line of defence. Whether you have an excruciating toothache, a 'slipped disc', a broken arm, or a flare up of a painful joint, painkillers can provide immediate relief to get you over the initial acute stage. Depending on your circumstances your physician may prescribe drugs over a longer period to control pain if it becomes chronic.

As I shall be showing in this chapter, other types of drug, which affect your mood, also have a role to play in reducing pain.

General guidelines for taking drugs

Before we look at what the various types of drugs do, I want first to make some important points about taking drugs of any description.

- Tell your doctor if you are taking any other drugs, since painkillers, or any drug for that matter, can produce side-effects when they interact with drugs already in your system – including alcohol.
- Tell your doctor about any side-effects or new symptoms as soon as possible after they occur. He may then decide to change you to another drug or reduce the dose.
- Never leave your pills where children can get hold of them. Some painkillers can easily be mistaken for sweets (candies).

- Don't take painkillers or other drugs if you are pregnant – or even if you only think you might be pregnant – before consulting your doctor. Some drugs can affect the healthy development of the foetus – especially in the first three months of pregnancy.
- If you find you need to take an over-the-counter painkiller for a new pain for more than three days, consult your doctor.
- Your doctor will prescribe the average dose to be taken at average times, and this will usually suit you, but not always. This means that you can use common sense in taking drugs a little more frequently – every three hours instead of every four, for instance – if they wear off more quickly than average. Conversely, if they are working well, you can extend the interval from, say, four hours to five. Please note that this does not apply to diabetics who must take their drugs at times specifically tailored for them. And no one should take twice as many pills in half the time!
- There are many names for each type of drug, so confusion is easy. Each drug has its chemical, or generic name, as well as a trade name. Throughout the book I refer to all drugs by their generic names, and to some, where appropriate also by some of their trade names, which are always written

with a capital first letter. Some drug names differ from country to country, so to avoid complicating the text I have included tables in this chapter and the Appendix which list the generic and some trade names of several drugs in different countries.

Simple painkillers (analgesics)

Aspirin is one of the best analgesic drugs that we have. It is available over the counter and is present in most households. Most people have used it at some time or other for headaches, the pains of bruises, period pain and toothache. Aspirin has four main benefits:

1. It relieves pain, and although only a mild analgesic it can relieve quite severe pain for a short time if a lot of it is taken. For instance, if you are on holiday, develop an agonizing toothache and cannot easily get to a dentist, taking two or three aspirins every four hours will help a great deal. Most people, though, cannot take aspirin in this quantity for more than a couple of days, as they become nauseated and may even vomit.
2. It reduces raised temperatures, and so is useful in treating fevers and infections.
3. It is an anti-prostaglandin drug, acting to reduce and eliminate the production of prostaglandins (see page 9) which cause particular pain in the rheumatic diseases and in painful periods.
4. It acts against inflammation, which is particularly useful in treating the rheumatic diseases such as arthritis.

Aspirin also has other advantages. For instance, it is very effective in reducing the ability of the blood to clot, and may be prescribed as a treatment to prevent stroke or coronary thrombosis (heart attack).

Side-effects Aspirin irritates the stomach lining and so should never be taken for abdominal pain, except gallstones (see pages 86–7). Regular doses of only one or two pills a day can cause bleeding in the stomach, and if this is large enough it may cause anaemia. Fortunately it does not do so in most people. Soluble aspirin compounds are a little easier on the stomach. Aspirin pills should always be taken with a liquid, and no aspirin should be taken whole on an empty stomach. In rare instances, large doses of aspirin can cause a severe and sometimes deadly condition – acidosis – in which the balance of acid and alkali in the blood is upset. Even mild poisoning with aspirin can cause buzzing in the ears and giddiness.

However, considering the huge amount taken (tonnes per week in Britain alone), there are not many side-effects if normal doses of one or two pills three times a day are taken for short periods. But I cannot repeat too often that what I say here is said in general terms and must never over-ride what your own personal physician says to you. After all, he or she knows your problems exactly, and if there are any doubts in your mind about anything I have said, mention it to your doctor and go by what is then said.

Other drugs There are other pills which have analgesic properties and also reduce temperature, but they are not anti-prostaglandins nor are they anti-inflammatory.

The best of these is paracetamol (acetaminophen in the United States). Like most drugs it has some side-effects, but taken in normal doses of two pills three or four times a day as a maximum, it is safe. If it is taken in excess, it can produce liver damage, and this is especially dangerous in children. But it does not irritate the stomach lining and so, unlike aspirin, can be used to treat some kinds of abdominal pain – peptic ulcers and gallstones, for example.

Benorylate (Benoral in Britain) is a compound of aspirin and paracetamol, which can be taken to relieve mild to moderate pain and to lower temperature. One dose can last up to eight hours. Its side-effects are more like aspirin's than paracetamol's, but it causes less irritation of the stomach than aspirin and the risk of liver damage with an overdose seems to be lower than with paracetamol.

A new prescription-only analgesic, about as powerful as paracetamol, is nefopam (Acupan in Britain). It is not fully understood how it works, but it may relieve moderate persistent pain that is unresponsive to other analgesics. Unlike aspirin and paracetamol, it does not lower temperature. In a few people it can cause nausea, and occasionally vomiting, and it should never be taken in combination with paracetamol due to the possible risk of damaging the liver.

Narcotics
Narcotics differ from simple analgesics in that, in addition to the pain-relieving properties, they also cause drowsiness and, in large doses, make you semi-conscious. Also unlike aspirin, paracetamol (acetaminophen) and nefopam, most narcotics are addictive, so very careful use must be made of them and they are only prescribed to those in really severe pain. Almost all the narcotics are based on or related to morphine which is extracted from opium.

Morphine produces pain relief, drowsiness, changes in mood and a reduction in mental activity; there is no complete loss of consciousness. The relief of pain is selective while other sensations – touch, hearing, sight – are unaffected. When proper doses are given, pain is still perceived, but the person does not seem to mind it. It makes breathing shallow and can produce violent vomiting in some people; also, it is well known for being very constipating. Its effect on breathing makes it unsuitable for anyone with a chest complaint, such as asthma or bronchitis.

The drugs in the table overleaf have the same effects as morphine to a greater or lesser degree.

Pethidine is a synthetic narcotic chemically dissimilar to morphine and is frequently used to relieve the pain of childbirth. Another common morphine-based drug, with a duration of four to five hours, is a combination of dextropropoxyphene and paracetamol (Distalgesic in Britain).

A very powerful synthetic narcotic that is said to be less addictive, and is thus suitable for relieving pain in conditions like post-herpetic neuralgia, is buprenorphine (Temgesic in Britain). It works best taken as small pellets that dissolve under the tongue and pain relief can last as long as twelve hours from one dose. It can cause vomiting in some people. Another strong narcotic with a very low risk of addiction is the recently introduced meptazinol (Meptid in Britain). This has the added benefit of having very little adverse effect on breathing. It is normally given by injection but pills have recently been developed. Again, some people do become a little nauseated.

Codeine, although derived from opium and officially classified as a narcotic, has little of the same action – in fact, it causes excitement rather than drowsiness – and in small doses, it can be taken as a simple analgesic for mild to moderate pain. It is also used in cough medicines and anti-diarrhoea preparations.

Morphine-type narcotics

Generic name & duration	UK trade name	Australia trade name	US trade name	Canada trade name
dextromoramide. 4 hours	Palfium	Palfium	Palfium	
dihydrocodeine 4 hours	DF118	Fortuss; Paracodin; Rikodeine	Paracodin	
dipipanone 4 hours	Diconal		Pipadone	
hydromorphone 4 hours	not available	Dilaudid	Dilaudid	Dilaudid
levorphanol 4 hours	Dromoran		Levo-Dromoran	Levo-Dromoran
pethidine } meperidine } 2–4 hours	Pethidine	Pethoid	Demerol	Demerol
methadone 3–5 hours	Physeptone	Physeptone	Dolophine	
oxymorphone 4 hours	not available		Numorphan	Numorphan
phenazocine 4 hours	Narphen	Narphen	Prinadol	

Pentazocine (Fortral in Britain) is a narcotic analgesic similar in action to codeine, but somewhat stronger, being prescribed for moderate to severe pain. Depending on the severity of the pain it may be given in pill form, by injection or by suppositories, and lasts up to four hours. It is not suitable for anyone with high blood pressure or for relieving the pain of heart failure.

Hypnotics
Hypnotic drugs are mainly prescribed to promote sleep; when small doses are given, the effect is simply to calm the emotions and then the drug is called a sedative. Hypnotics have no effect on the cause of pain itself, but they do reduce accompanying anxiety and agitation, and can allow sleep when previously this may have been impossible, and so can affect your pain tolerance.

Barbiturates have been largely replaced by other, safer drugs because of their side-effects, and their use as a sleep-inducer against insomnia caused by pain is very limited. These drugs are all addictive. They also slow down the rate of breathing, reduce blood pressure and lower the body temperature, the latter being particularly dangerous in the elderly. They can markedly speed up the liver processes, which can make them interact badly with other drugs. Taking them causes drowsiness and this can have a bad hangover effect – the person using barbiturates to sleep will feel the effects long after waking in the morning, and driving cars and operating machinery should be avoided. The effect of barbiturates can lead to 'drug automatism': a person taking them wakes in a daze, thinks he needs more of the drug and

Barbiturates

Generic name	UK trade name	Australia trade name	US trade name	Canada trade name
amylobarbitone amylobarbital	Amytal	Amytal	Amytal	Amytal
butabarbital butobarbitone	Soneryl	Butisol; Soneryl	Butisol Sodium	Day-Barb; Soneryl
methohexitone methohexital (anaesthesia)	Brietal Sodium	Brietal Sodium	Brevital Sodium	Brietal Sodium
pentobarbitone pentobarbital	Nembutal	Nembutal	Nembutal	Nembutal
quinalbarbitone secobarbital	Seconal Sodium	Seconal Sodium	Seconal Sodium	Seconal Sodium
thiopentone thiopental (anaesthesia)	Intraval Sodium	Pentothal Sodium	Pentothal	Pentothal Sodium

takes an overdose by mistake.

Because of the above and other side-effects, barbiturates are now mainly used only as short-acting general anaesthetics in dentistry and other types of surgery, and for very severe insomnia when nothing else works.

Benzodiazepines Like barbiturates, these reduce the anxiety, agitation and tension that often accompany and aggravate pain, but they are not nearly so physically addictive, although there is growing evidence of psychological dependence. Fatal overdoses, though, are very rare. They are widely used, with more than 30 million prescriptions written annually in Britain alone. In the context of pain relief, I often prescribe them when acute pain is making it particularly hard for a patient to get to sleep. To avoid the problem of possible dependence, they should be taken only for a short period of time – a week or so – just to get you over a bad patch. Because they make you feel dopey and wobbly-kneed, you should not drive a car or operate heavy machinery while taking benzodiazepines.

Alcohol is a drug that has a definite sedative effect, and before the advent of modern drugs was one of the only available 'painkillers'. Many people today drink alcohol to help them relax and go to sleep, and you might think its effects make it an ideal aid to pain relief. In fact, research has shown that although alcohol gets you off to sleep quicker, it has a rebound effect which disturbs your sleep later on in the night. Also, drinking substantial amounts of alcohol to help you with the pain can become a dangerous habit, as alcohol is a physically addictive drug. In short, I believe it has but a small role to play in relieving pain.

Antidepressants

Tricyclics Your doctor may prescribe tricyclic antidepressants if you are both depressed and anxious about your pain. These drugs are called 'tricyclic' be-

Benzodiazepines

Generic name	UK trade name	Australia trade name	US trade name	Canada trade name
chlordiaze-poxide	Librium; Tropium	Librium	A-Poxide; Librium; SK-Lygen	Librium; Medilium; Relaxil; Solium
clobazam	Frisium	not available	not available	not available
clorazepate dipotassium	Tranxene	Tranxene	Tranxene	Tranxene
diazepam	Atensine; Evacalm; Solis; Valium	Ducene; Pro-Pam; Valium	Valium	Meval; Neo-Calme; Rival; Valium; Vivol
flurazepam	Dalmane	Dalmane	Dalmane	Dalmane; Novoflupam; Somnol; Som-Pam
ketazolam	Anxon	not available	not available	Loftran
lorazepam	Ativan	Ativan	Ativan	Ativan
lormetazepam	Noctamid	not available	not available	not available
medazepam	Nobrium	no longer available	not available	not available
nitrazepam	Mogadon; Nitrados; Somnite; Surem	Dormicum; Mogadon	not available	Mogadon
temazepam	Euhypnos; Normison	Euhypnos; Normison	Restoril	Restoril
triazolam	Halcion	not available	not available	Halcion

cause originally their molecular structure contained three rings. They may take as long as two to three weeks before they relax you, improve your appetite and the quality of your sleep (so that other hypnotics may not be necessary). Antidepressants are not addictive, but they do have troublesome, rather than serious, side-effects which may include drowsiness, a dry mouth, blurred vision, sweating and constipation.

MAOIs You may be prescribed another type of antidepressant called a monoamine oxidase inhibitor (MAOI, for short), which stops the development of certain chemicals that excite the brain. Great care must be taken to avoid certain food and drinks when on MAOIs – meat and yeast extracts, cheese, alcohol, canned fish and so on – because they can react with these drugs, causing dangerously high blood pressure which is first noticed as a throbbing headache.

Analgesics, narcotics, hypnotics and antidepressants can prove useful when

Tricyclic antidepressants

Generic name	UK trade name	Australia trade name	US trade name	Canada trade name
amitriptyline	Domical; Lentizol, Saroten; Tryptizol	Amitrip; Laroxyl; Tryptanol; Saroten	Amitid; Elavil; Endep	Deprex; Elavil; Levate; Meravil; Novotriptyn
butriptyline	Evadyne	not available	not available	not available
clomipramine	Anafranil	not available	not available	Anafranil
desipramine	Pertofran	Pertofran	Norpramin; Pertofrane	Norpramin; Pertofrane
dothiepin	Prothiaden	Prothiaden	not available	not available
doxepin	Sinequan	Quitaxon; Sinequan	Adapin; Sinequan	Sinequan
imipramine	Tofranil	Imiprin; Iramil; Prodepress; Tofranil	Janimine; SK-Pramine; Tofranil	Impril; Novopramine; Tofranil
iprindole	Prondol	not available	not available	not available
nortriptyline	Allegron; Aventyl	Allegron; Nortab	Aventyl; Pamelor	Aventyl
protriptyline	Concordin	Concordin	Vivactil	Triptil
trimipramine	Surmontil	Surmontil	Surmontil	Surmontil

MAOIs

Generic name	UK trade name	Australia trade name	US trade name	Canada trade name
iproniazid	Marsilid	Marsilid	not available	not available
isocarboxazid	Marplan	Marplan	Marplan	Marplan
phenelzine	Nardil	Nardil	Nardil	Nardil
tranylcypromine	Parnate	Parnate	Parnate	Parnate

prescribed for specific conditions for limited periods. You also need to learn to cope with your pain and its attendant stress, anxiety and depression in the long term, and the non-drug methods which I have outlined in Chapters 11 and 12 may help a great deal with this.

Anaesthetics

The main purpose of anaesthetics is to eliminate pain from surgical operations, including dental procedures. They are also used for pain relief – in childbirth for example. There are different types of anaesthetics, but they all work by approximately the same method. They either stop nerves from transmitting electrical impulses or they block these impulses in the spinal cord or brain. This prevents the transmission of all sorts of functions – sensation, movement, and so forth – but particularly the transmission of pain, and there is also sometimes a loss of consciousness. They are divided into two main groups: the general anaesthetics and the local anaesthetics.

General anaesthetics

These are given by injection into a vein or are breathed in, and they have a direct effect on the nerve cells of the brain so that you lose consciousness. The skill of giving anaesthetics is to give you exactly enough for you to lose consciousness and to allow your muscles to relax so that surgery can be carried out.

Ether, chloroform, trilene and halothane are powerful general anaesthetics which are inhaled. Nitrous oxide – 'laughing gas' – is a weaker one which is often used in dental treatment and with oxygen to help the pain of the contractions during childbirth (see page 82); it is also sometimes used in combination with one of the other inhaled anaesthetics. Injections of one of the strong, quick-acting barbiturates (see pages 94–5) are also given.

Before a general anaesthetic is used, you are usually given 'premedication'. This may include small doses of any of the narcotics or hypnotics already mentioned to calm and relax you, as well as a drug which reduces salivation, to prevent you from inhaling saliva.

Side-effects   A major problem during a general anaesthetic is that, as all your muscles relax, so do the jaw muscles and therefore the jaw and the tongue tend to obstruct your breathing. Anaesthetists (anaesthesiologists in the United States) have many devices for preventing this happening, from just holding up the jaw with their hands to putting a plastic airway into the mouth which you can breathe through. In long and involved operations, a special tracheal tube is inserted through the mouth and into the windpipe (trachea) so that there is no chance of you not being able to breathe.

Local anaesthetics

These are given when a relatively small area of the body needs to be anaesthetized, such as a finger to have an abscess opened up, or when a general anaesthetic is considered to be unsuitable. If the anaesthetist (anaesthesiologist) wishes to prevent all sensation from a given part of the body reaching your brain, a local anaesthetic can be injected into the nerves supplying, say, the whole of the abdomen before an abdominal operation, or a whole hip in a hip replacement. In such major operations, you are usually not kept awake, but are put into a light sleep with a small dose of a general anaesthetic so that you cannot remember anything of the procedure.

A local anaesthetic injected into the epidural space surrounding the spinal cord is often used in childbirth. This is discussed on pages 82–3. Local anaesthetics in the form of gels may also be rubbed on a painful area or sprayed on; this last is frequently used by athletes during competitions.

The length of time that a local anaesthetic lasts depends on the type used. There are short-lasting anaesthetics and long-lasting ones, varying between

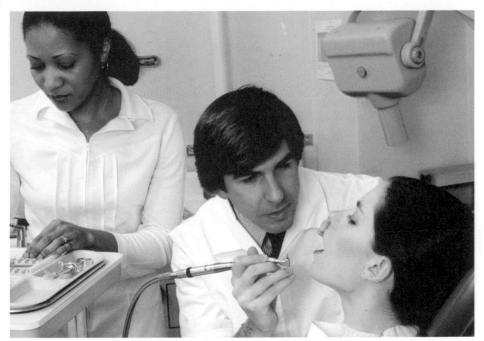
Local anaesthetics help to make modern dental treatment a pain-free experience.

thirty minutes and five hours.

Dental treatment The place where most local anaesthetics are used, with tremendous expertise, is in dental treatment. Millions of people throughout the world are given local anaesthetics each year with enormous safety, thus avoiding problems with breathtaking, alterations in blood pressure and unconsciousness which can occur with a general anaesthetic.

When a dentist uses local anaesthesia to 'freeze' the teeth, he can do it in one of two ways. He can inject the drug near the root of an individual tooth so that only that tooth becomes numb, or he can inject it near a nerve which is supplying a number of teeth so that the whole of the lower jaw or the upper jaw on one side is affected. The benefit of this type of injection is that, as it is made into a confined space – the gum near a nerve root – the local anaesthetic is very concentrated and the effect takes

place exceedingly quickly. Often the whole or a part of the tongue is also affected by the anaesthetic, and can remain numb for a while after leaving the dentist. Until sensation returns, it is very important to make a conscious effort not to bite your tongue.

Side-effects Occasionally, as with any other type of treatment, there is a patient who reacts badly to a local anaesthetic, and this is usually because he or she has an allergy to the drug used. There is very little that can be done about this except to treat the reaction when it occurs and for the patient to avoid the drug in the future. But apart from this, local anaesthesia is an exceedingly safe method.

Anaesthesia and drugs are not, of course, the only methods of pain relief. In the next chapter I shall be describing other ways in which medical professionals can help you to conquer your pain.

11. NON-DRUG METHODS OF PAIN RELIEF

Electrical stimulation therapy: rubbing it better

The role of the two types of nerve fibres – the thin C fibres and the thicker A-beta fibres – has already been discussed in Chapter 1. The C fibres carry only pain, but the large A-beta fibres also have quite a lot to do with the way you feel pain. These are able to block the signals of pain that pass along the thin C fibres towards the brain and your consciousness, and they do this in the spinal cord in a way that is not fully understood called gate control. What seems to happen is that, when the skin is damaged, both small and large nerve fibres are stimulated and send information to the spinal cord. There, the faster, non-painful stimulation from the large A fibres prevents some of the slower, painful stimulation from the small C fibres from passing on.

Your own unconscious plays a part in this. When you hurt yourself by, say, knocking a hip against the corner of a table, you automatically rub the sore part. What you are doing is increasing the stimulation along the large A fibres and this travels to the spinal cord where it blocks more of the painful stimulation travelling at a slower rate along the C fibres. You do not have to be taught to do this as it is an automatic action; even very young children do it after they have fallen over, and anybody who has had any dealings with children will know the value of 'rubbing it better'.

As soon as the scientists realized the way in which rubbing worked in relieving pain, they set about producing an artificial method of doing the same thing. It was found that a painful region could be stimulated by a small electric current (produced by a special apparatus) passing through the skin between small carbon-rubber conduction pads – called electrodes – placed on the skin. This method, which has been widely available for the last ten years, is known as transcutaneous electrical nerve stimulation and is usually abbreviated to TENS.

What sort of pain can TENS relieve? Any type of pain may respond to TENS and therefore it should always be tried, but the technique does stand a better chance if the pain is not terribly severe. In other words, it often works best for pain of medium intensity, and I have found that it also performs better in pains which are fairly constant – such as headache, stiff neck, backache, bruises, fractures which have been set, and sometimes period pain – rather than in the 'shooting' varieties, as in the pain caused by blood vessel disease (see Chapter 5). Another condition for which it is often not successful is post-herpetic neuralgia – the nerve pain after shingles that mostly affects elderly people (see Chapter 9). Shingles destroys some of the large A-beta nerve fibres, leaving mostly, and sometimes only, the thin C fibres that carry pain. If a painful area occurs where there are few A-beta nerve endings in the skin, then there is little for the apparatus to stimulate in order to reduce pain. In a few people with post-herpetic neuralgia all the A-beta fibres are destroyed, and for them TENS will not work, as there is nothing for it to work on. Despite this problem, my advice with post-herpetic neuralgia – and any other type of pain – is try TENS and see.

In some hospitals, TENS is used after certain operations to reduce the pain from wounds, particularly in chest operations and some abdominal ones. By using this method, it is possible to reduce the amount of painkillers needed or eliminate them completely. The problem here is to place electrodes along the edges of the wound and still keep the wound sterile so that infection cannot arise. A special type of aluminium foil electrode has been developed that can be placed along the edges of wounds, using a special adhesive; its great advantage is that it can be sterilized easily.

TENS has also been safely and successfully used in childbirth, but some women have found it difficult to keep the electrodes in place and a few have developed an allergic skin reaction to the electrodes. If you want to use TENS during labour it is wise to practise with it beforehand to help anticipate any problems that may occur.

How effective is it? TENS works for about 10 per cent of those who try it. Although TENS tends to reduce pain and not cut it out entirely, it *is* possible for it to relieve a pain completely. But the stronger the pain is to start with, the less chance there is of a perfect result. Don't forget that your own rubbing does not get rid of all the pain – it only helps it – but this amount of help may make all the difference between not needing heavy medication and needing it, or being able to go to work and not being able to do so.

For many people, the relieving or elimination of pain sometimes lasts up to three or four times as long as the original stimulation, but for most, the relief continues only while the stimulation is occurring.

Using the apparatus The apparatus must be prescribed by your doctor and you will usually have to buy it (some are available on the National Health Service in Britain, but these are in short supply). However, most of the companies who offer them for sale will give you two-thirds of your money back if you find that it does not work for you. But do make sure of this before buying. Some hospital physiotherapy departments may be able to loan you one for a trial.

An added bonus is that the TENS apparatus can be obtained in very small, pocket-sized versions which can be concealed in clothing. A larger type – but still small enough for a pocket – is also available, the batteries of which last the length of the working day before needing changing. The very small machines cost about as much as a cheap colour television; the larger pocket-size ones are comparable in price to a good quality transistor radio. There are many people walking about today using TENS, and their friends and workmates do not even known about it.

When you use one of these devices – and there are many different makes of them – you will feel a tingling through your skin and into the painful region. If the pads are over or near one of the large nerves in the skin, the tingling may spread along that nerve into another part of the body. Thus, if the pads are placed at the top of your leg, the tingling may spread down the sciatic nerve towards your toes.

The best placing of the pads to obtain relief is largely a matter of trial and error. To start with put them on very close to the painful region and if that is not successful, try other positions.

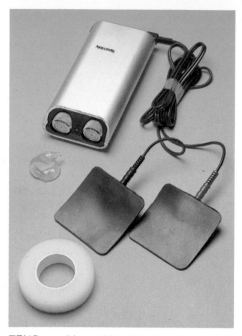

TENS machine with adhesive tape and contact gel for the pads.

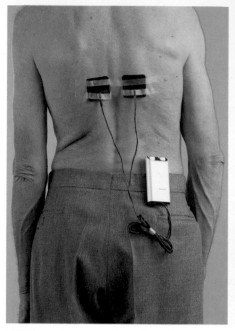

TENS machine set up for backache.

If you have a particularly tender area on your back, say, place the pads around it rather than on it. For tension headache, the best position for the pads is often on each side of the back of the neck; and for period pain, just above the pubic bone below your tummy, or on the haunches on either side of the spine at hip level.

TENS is not dangerous, but as with any machine used for a medical purpose, your doctor will show you how to use it properly or arrange for this to be done.

Naturally, this electrical apparatus, must be used with common sense so that you do not turn the power control up so high that it hurts. Special care must be taken if you have patches of numbness or decreased sensitivity on your skin, because you can turn up the power without it hurting and may damage your skin. There is never any point in turning up the power high, as TENS only works if the tingling sen-sation is gentle and reaches the spinal cord to stop pain getting through.

There are a few other obvious precautions to take. It is inadvisable to use this in the first three months of pregnancy, and some doctors say that it should not be used at all during pregnancy. Some people's skin is sensitive to the gel used between the electrodes and the skin to make good electrical contact. If your skin under the pads becomes a little reddened or uncomfortable, stop using the device and contact the doctor who prescribed it. The apparatus can also affect the operation of some types of heart pacemakers and those who have these, as well as those who suffer from any disease affecting the heart's rhythm, should not use TENS. The area around the eye and the eye itself should never be stimulated, and you should never abruptly increase the amount of stimulation while operating dangerous machinery or driving.

Acupuncture

Acupuncture has been used in China for at least 4,000 years, and there it has developed into a common method of medical treatment, particularly for pain. In fact, most pain relief clinics elsewhere in the world now use it. In certain countries such as France (where 10 per cent of hospitals have departments of acupuncture), the technique can only be carried out by qualified medical doctors, while in most other countries, non-medical practitioners as well as doctors provide it.

How does it work? The Chinese doctors who first used acupuncture tried to explain how it worked in terms of the science of that time. They believed that the universe is filled with a life force – *Chi* – and part of this life force is in every living thing. In humans, it circulates around the body in channels called meridians which are connected to various organs in the body – the heart, lungs, liver and so on. The flow of *Chi* is influenced by the forces of *Yin* and *Yang* which roughly correspond to 'negative' and 'positive' or 'female' and 'male'. When *Yin* and *Yang* (and, with them, the flow of the life force in the meridians) become unbalanced, disease results. According to this system, the affected meridians can be picked out by feeling the patient's pulse at the wrist in a special fashion. By placing a solid acupuncture needle at a certain point on the meridians, the balance of *Yin* and *Yang* and the flow of *Chi* can be corrected and health results.

Today, many – particularly non-medical – practitioners carry out the whole ancient regime without change. However, scientists have done much research into how acupuncture works and, although much of it still remains a mystery, a good part of it can now be explained.

Many acupuncture points are over places where nerves come through the deep tissues towards the skin and therefore are sensitive places where nerves can be affected. Other acupuncture points are placed over or near motor nerve end-plates – that is, where the nerve to a muscle enters the muscle. Thus any stimulation at these places has a profound effect on the nervous system. In addition, 71 per cent of traditional acupuncture points correspond to what are known as 'trigger points' – small areas on the skin which become tender during certain diseases. The referred pain (see page 12) of heart disease, where it is felt in the shoulder, is one example, but many others do not have any noticeable nerve connection with the cause of the pain.

In acupuncture, the pain is usually relieved by the manipulation of the inserted needle. Modern science has shown that this stimulation by an acupuncture needle will increase the production of chemicals called endorphins, which are the body's own

Acupuncture to relieve migraine.

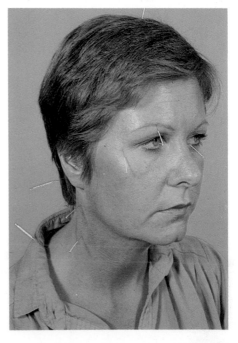

natural painkillers. But there are probably many other mechanisms at work, since the stimulation of a painful area is, as we have seen, the principle behind gate control and TENS therapy (pages 10 and 100–2), and the production of an alternate, milder pain is the basis of counter-irritants (pages 112–13); an element of distracting the mind (pages 15–16) is also involved.

Clearly, there is some way to go before we fully understand how acupuncture works, as no one has explained scientifically how the technique exerts its effect over long periods of time. At present research is being conducted into this question. In 1980 Dr Ronald Katz in the US showed that in certain patients chronic pain could be cured by painful daily stimulation of the nerves for up to a year with a technique very similar to acupuncture.

How acupuncture is performed
There are three principal techniques of using acupuncture needles. The first gives a brief, very strong stimulation to the patient, which is usually painful. The needle is inserted and twisted backwards and forwards vigorously, providing an intense stimulation for about five to ten seconds. Another method is to insert a needle or, more usually, a number of them and leave them in for about twenty or thirty minutes. This should not be painful. Sometimes these needles are connected to an apparatus which passes a mild, usually painless electric current through them for about fifteen to twenty minutes. Thirdly, the acupuncturist will search out the tender 'trigger points' on a patient's body, and insert a needle into each. This takes considerable time because the entire skin has to be examined. Whichever of these techniques is used, when the needle enters the right spot, a numb sensation spreads around the needle, often tingling along the nerve.

Some of these same techniques can be learned and used by anyone, but using acu*pressure* instead of needles. In this, you press your fingers on certain sites where nerves approach the surface of the skin. The Chinese have developed this into a sophisticated system called *Shiatsu*, but a simpler technique can be found in the many books available on the subject which have been published in recent years.

How effective is acupuncture?
There are, of course, all sorts of claims for acupuncture – that it will cure all sorts of diseases – but the only evidence we have so far for its value is that it is useful in relieving painful conditions – doctors have reported a 70 per cent success rate in treating arthritis, migraine and period pains.

In those people for whom acupuncture is successful, the pain relief lasts much longer than the time the needles are in the skin. The length of time varies from person to person. But in my hospital, where acupuncture is used to treat migraine in patients for whom normal treatment by drugs has not worked, two-thirds of those who respond well to acupuncture get relief from headaches for at least one month after a twenty-minute session. If each treatment does relieve the pain for a month, then twelve treatments a year – the maximum number I would recommend – can keep a patient reasonably free from pain.

Mostly the migraine is not cured by using this technique, but only improved. Of course, most patients who have had very severe migraine every week for two or more days are quite satisfied with this.

Acupuncture has also been used successfully during childbirth, although in my own region it has not proved as effective as TENS. It has also been used for dental treatment and as an anaesthetic for surgical operations. The latter is not as successful as the others, some doctors saying that it is only completely effective in 5 to 10 per cent of cases. However, it can sometimes be used in combination with other forms of anaesthesia (see pages 98–9) and may help reduce the amount of drugs that need to be taken.

In general, acupuncture can be used for any painful condition, it is not a difficult procedure to carry out and there is little risk attached to it as long as the needles are properly sterilized. If they are not, the patient may develop infective hepatitis, abscesses or other blood-borne types of infection that are present in the previous patients on whom the needles were used. But remember that acupuncture cannot help with any disease in which there has been actual tissue damage – in other words, it cannot knit broken bones and cannot cure cancer, heart disease or any other similar condition. It can often relieve the pain caused by these, but this can lead to problems as, by masking the pain, you may delay having its cause diagnosed and treated. This is one of the major reasons for never going to a non-medically qualified acupuncturist. To reach an acupuncturist who is also a doctor, ask your family doctor if he or she can refer you to one, or get in touch with one of the organizations listed on pages 114–16.

Hypnosis

We do not fully understand how hypnosis works. Essentially, it involves you allowing a hypnotist to relax you into a type of trance and, while you are in this relaxed state, to give you suggestions which can have great impact and effect.

Not everybody can be hypnotized. Only 5 per cent of the population can be placed in a deep trance easily; others can do so after a number of sessions and most of us are able to pass into light trances, but a few cannot be hypnotized at all. The problem in hypnosis, though, is not in getting you into a trance, but in having enough skill to bring you out of the relaxed state in a proper way so that you behave perfectly normally afterwards. In Europe, hypnosis as a stage act was banned following one occasion when a stage hypnotist was unable to bring a subject out satisfactorily. Thus hypnosis and hypnotherapy must be given by competent, qualified practitioners. As with acupuncturists, ask your family doctor to recommend one or contact one of the organizations given on pages 114–16.

Hypnosis has mainly been used to help treat certain psychological problems, as it often enables you to uncover buried conflicts and problems or recall forgotten emotional experiences. As it induces a feeling of well-being and relaxation in most people and can sometimes have an anaesthetic effect, it has also been used for the relief of pain of many types, up to and including that of severe cancer pain. It will relieve pain in a small proportion of patients, and figures given for this vary between 5 and 10 per cent. The people who are hypnotized very easily are often the ones who can obtain pain relief by this method. In the past, I have used hypnosis to allow a patient to have crowns fitted to the upper front teeth without any local anaesthetic being required. Normally this is quite a painful process, as the teeth have first to be cut down in size before the crowns are fitted on top of them.

In summary I would say that hypnosis is a method which can be tried for chronic pain, and like many fringe treatments may work when other methods have failed. But before you have to turn to hypnosis as a last resort, there are many simple but effective ways of alleviating pain that you can do yourself, and I shall be describing these in the next chapter.

12. SELF-HELP

Rest and relaxation

If you are in pain you may become nervous about what is going to happen to you. You may wonder whether you are ever going to get rid of the pain which is present night and day, and you are naturally anxious about when you will be able to return to your job and home, and whether your life-style is going to suffer because your income may drop both while you are ill and when you are recovering.

Not only are you anxious but you may become depressed as well – and quite understandably so. Your pulse rate increases, you look worried and your whole personality may change. Pain is increased under these circumstances: your pain tolerance level falls and you become more sensitive to pain. Thus a continuous circle is set up – pain produces anxiety and depression, which reduces resistance to pain and this produces more anxiety and depression.

Broken bones are placed in splints or plaster to rest them. Migraine sufferers lie down in a quiet darkened room until the attack is over. An acute attack of a rheumatic disease or a strained or torn muscle demand rest until the acute episode is over and any swelling and spasm of the muscles have settled down. The body as a whole also needs rest and sleep, to recoup the strength it has lost due to the strain of a disease and the pain that it has brought.

If only you could relax, you could achieve this rest much more easily and be more capable of coping with your pain by breaking the vicious circle I have just described. Just how much you would benefit from this is difficult to say; it depends on the type of personality you had before the illness. Some people are born worriers, others have built-in optimism. You cannot expect your personality to change with rest and relaxation, only that you may return to the way you were before.

Relaxation does not only help to cope with the pain of an illness such as arthritis. Anxiety caused, for example, by childbirth or a dental operation, will tense up the muscles and aggravate the pain. Relaxation is a well-tried method of reducing or at least taking the edge off pain that is made worse by tension.

Relaxation methods that are taught

There are now many methods of relaxation that are taught, and one of the reasons for the success of some of them is that it seems to be easier to relax if somebody else is giving you instructions. Whichever method is used, there is one essential – you have to be taught to relax all your muscles. Doing this under hypnosis is probably the quickest way, but there are some people who cannot be treated successfully in this way, and in any case, a hypnotherapist is required (see previous chapter). An alternative is to study meditation or yoga, where the initial requirement is to produce a state of relaxation. Autogenic therapy is also taught and involves learning how to talk to your body, to make it relax virtually on command.

It is always easier to continue with a method if you have first been shown how to do it. Some systems will also provide you with tapes of an instructor's voice which can be played when you relax on your own, and this can be a very successful method. Biofeedback (see page 70) can also be used with relaxation exercises, to give you an idea as to how you are progressing and to give a goal to achieve – that is, the reduction in the bleeps that are heard or the flashing light which indicates that the body is relaxing.

DIY relaxation If you have to rely on your own efforts, the following will give you the basic ideas of most relaxation techniques. Lie down somewhere where you are comfortable and warm; it is no use trying to relax if you are cold and uncomfortable. If your pain is such that you are more comfortable lying flat on the floor with one pillow, then use that position.

Close your eyes, concentrate and think about your face, unless that is where your pain is; if that is the case, think of somewhere that is not painful, say, your foot. No matter which part of your body you concentrate on, the technique is the same – to go mentally over the muscles of that part, one by one, and consciously relax them.

In your face, think of the muscles around your mouth and let them go loose – then your cheeks, followed by those around your eyes and the back of your head. They should feel so loose that they almost slip off your face on to the pillow. At first, it is difficult but do the best you can and then go on to relax the muscles of your neck. These are in four groups at the right and left front and the right and left back. So, one by one, think of each of these and

Taking time out to go through a relaxation routine can help take the edge off pain that's made worse by anxious tension.

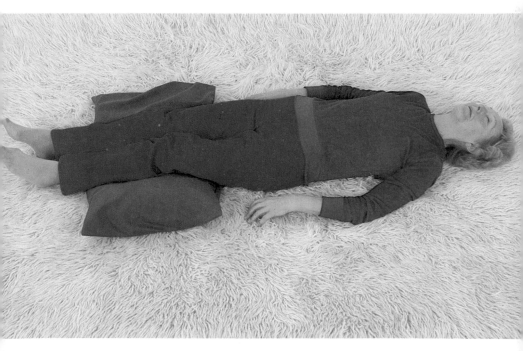

consciously make them relax – the front right muscles, the front left ones, the back left ones and finally the back right ones. You do not have to do them in any particular order – just please yourself.

Now make sure that you are still lying comfortably. No lumps under you? The pillow nicely smoothed? Are you warm enough? Concentrate on your breathing. Try to do this slowly and deeply, and every time you breathe out, make a mental effort to relax the muscles in your chest, back and abdomen. After breathing steadily for a few minutes, you will gradually realize that, however sceptical you were to start with, you are actually loosening up.

Return to your face muscles (or those in your foot or wherever) and go over them once again. Then back to the breathing and relax your body some more. Go on down the rest of it, relaxing your bottom so that your pelvis flops on the floor or the bed, then your thighs, calves and feet. Next concentrate on your arms, first relaxing your shoulders, then your upper arms, your lower arms and your hands.

While all this is going on, at another level of your mind you can tell yourself that you are breathing more slowly, that your muscles are relaxing and that you are feeling more comfortable. Also tell yourself that, if you go off to sleep (you may become so comfortable that you will sleep for five minutes or so) when you wake up you will feel refreshed and relaxed. It is important to make sure that you tell yourself that you will feel perfectly relaxed both mentally and physically, whether you wake up yourself or somebody else does it: you do not want to wake up with a start.

Essentially that is all that relaxation is about. Once you get used to it, the relaxation takes place rapidly, and it can be used during the day whenever you have a quiet moment, to give yourself a boost. After a time, you will notice that you are using the method during everyday life without really being aware of it, lessening tension and reducing your pain.

Exercise

Gentle exercise is a well-known way of improving a painful condition, such as an arthritic joint or a stiff neck, after an initial period of rest. It is a fact that if muscles or joints are rested and not moved through their full range for a time, due to acute pain – or for any other reason – the muscles become thin and wasted and the joints become stiff. If you then try to exercise them even in the gentlest of ways, the muscles stiffen and ache and the joints become sore. Although the scale is different, the result is exactly comparable to the stiffness and soreness that an athlete gets when he or she begins to train again at the beginning of the season after a layoff.

Unfortunately, this discomfort may make you feel that your body is warning you that you are doing too much and so you return to inactivity. This is exactly the wrong thing to do in most cases, as gentle, graduated exercises are often the way to start you back on the road to recovery and a relatively normal life. The graduated exercises needed for this type of programme are best obtained from a qualified physiotherapist, who will design a programme with your medical history in mind and will work together with your medical advisor.

There are four reasons why exercise is important after a period of enforced inactivity:

1. To help prevent long-term pain and stiffness in muscles and joints caused by lack of movement.
2. To strengthen the muscles to increase their power and also to

provide endurance and stability (for example, to stabilize the spine).

3. To mobilize the body by providing a full range of movement in the various joints and combinations of joints (such as that found in leaning backwards).
4. To maintain and improve the working of the joints.

Graduated exercises must be planned on an individual basis. If one of my patients has been bedridden with a painful condition for two months, it is no use immediately prescribing a brisk walk each morning. During the first day or two, such patients will walk to the bedside armchair two or three times a day; all doctors try to ensure that their patients get out of bed each day – even if it is only for a few minutes. The patients will also get some mild physiotherapy to their legs, especially for those muscles on the front of the thighs – the vasti muscles – which support us when we stand. The physiotherapist will try to exercise these muscles by lifting and bending exercises when the patients are confined to bed but are not too ill. If you are in bed for any length of time, your thighs become obviously thin. I usually reckon that a week in bed needs one month of exercise to get these vasti muscles back to their old strength and size, while a month of bedrest takes them three months to do the same thing.

It is important always to go through the complete range of any movement and it is usually the last bit of the action which will do the most good. For example, if you are asked to extend your neck (to lift your head as high up off your shoulders as possible), you must do so as *fully* as you can, not just 95 per cent of the way. Similarly, if you are asked to straighten your elbow, you must really straighten the joint, getting those last few degress of movement. It is vital, though, that you check to find out whether you should exercise freely before undertaking a course of instruction. That is why the help of a trained physiotherapist is so important.

Preventing pain with regular exercise Many people feel that, because they move about – walking, bending, going up and down stairs – while carrying out their normal activities, that is enough to keep their muscles and joints supple and pain free, but it is not. They are using only a limited number of movements and these are not taken to the fullest extent. A full range of body movements, and individual exercises for any part of the body that may have limited movement because of painful injury or disease, are all necessary on a regular basis.

Posture (see page 44) is important to preserve the proper relationships between the various joints and bones and to prevent the painful straining of ligaments and joints by bad alignment. Thus posture exercises and free movement are often done together, and such activities as dancing, swimming and 'musical movement' (exercising to music) are very useful in this respect. It is important to go to a properly trained teacher – a dancer will teach dance movement very well but may not recognize the joint limitations of old or ill people. Yoga is very worth while but, again, you must be capable of making the movements. Imagine trying to get mobility into the hip of an elderly person (perhaps only a few years away from a hip replacement operation): it would be quite impossible and could only make matters worse. The important thing to remember is that care must be taken and common sense used.

It is quite impossible to give exercises for all eventualities – that is why we have physiotherapists – but if you are

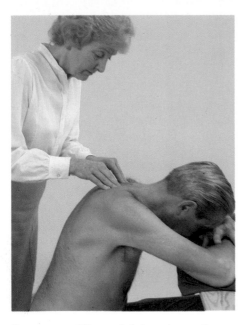

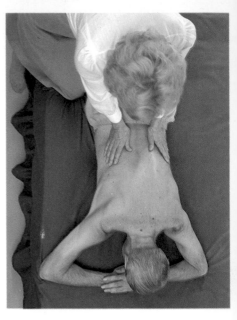

To ease a stiff or painful neck, gently knead the muscles on either side of the spine and at the top of the shoulders.

Gentle circular massage can do wonders for a tense, painful back. Be careful not to touch the spine.

The warmth from a material-covered hot-water bottle can be very soothing for stomach-ache or period pain.

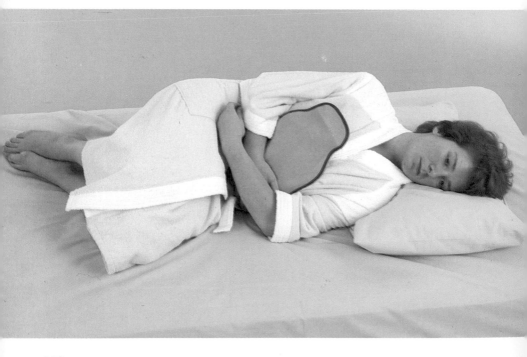

in good health, you should run through a series of exercises every day to make sure that you maintain a full range of movement in all of your joints. The following exercises appear in the relevant chapters earlier in this book:

- Neck and head (page 32)
- Shoulders and arms (page 33)
- Spine and back (page 52)
- Legs (page 35)

Doing these exercises for a total of fifteen to twenty minutes each day is quite enough. Remember to be reasonable when starting: do three of each for a few days, then five, adding on one or two each week until ten is reached.

In my experience, this type of exercise creates a mood of well-being, and mood, as we have seen, plays a great part in the way you are affected by pain. An optimistic and positive approach through exercise can work wonders for morale and your pain.

Massage

Massage can also be used to keep limbs mobile and reduce pain. Not only does it increase the blood supply to the muscles and tissues that are stimulated by the massage, prevent wasting, relax tense muscles and promote a feeling of well-being, but by stimulating the A-beta nerves in the skin it also produces a pain-relieving effect by gate control, similar to 'rubbing it better' and TENS therapy (see previously in this chapter).

If it is possible to go to a trained masseur or physiotherapist, this is the best course. But in many cases this is not possible on a daily basis, and in the interim, your spouse, relatives or friends can help. Gentle kneading of the shoulder and neck muscles is easy to do, and is marvellously soothing for a splitting headache or stiff neck. This type of gentle movement of other muscles and joints can be performed by those who have not been specially trained (see illustrations opposite). Massage can be tried for any type of pain and can be done anywhere in the body as long as it is remembered both that if the person who is being massaged feels pain, this is a sign that the amateur massage is too vigorous, and that the spine itself should never be touched. Talc, baby oil or a pain-relieving liniment (see page 113) can be used to reduce friction.

Do not imagine that this can be a full substitute for the regular professional treatment – it cannot – but it can be soothing and should enable you to have easier movement of your joints.

Heat treatment

Warmth is useful in helping just about every type of pain. The hot-water bottle against the skin is a well-known remedy for an ache or pain. Obvious care must be taken not to burn the skin and the simplest ways of avoiding this are, first, never to fill the bottle with boiling water; second, never to overfill it; and third, to make sure that all of its surface is covered (and stays covered) so that none of the rubber can come into contact with the skin. There is a special danger of scalds or burns when heat is used on children, so extra care must be taken. A small electric heating pad is perhaps safer for both children and adults. Both hot-water bottles and heating pads should be applied to the painful area for fifteen to twenty minutes several times a day, as needed.

There are two theories about why heat treatment is effective in reducing pain. First, the heat increases the diameters of the blood vessels and thus increases the blood flow. This means that healing agents – chemicals and other substances – can get to a damaged area quicker, and harmful products – such as kinins and prostaglandins (see pages 9 and 79) – can be swept away. Second, the heat may stimulate the nerves in the skin in much the same way that the electrical impulses in

TENS therapy (pages 100–2) do, thus changing your perception of pain.

Other variations of heat treatment have been used for centuries by different cultures: Roman baths, Japanese hot soaking tubs, Russian and Turkish steam rooms, Scandinavian saunas. In addition, doctors and physiotherapists make use of two forms of mechanically created heat. Ultrasound therapy uses very high frequencies of sound (over one million cycles per second) which cannot be heard by the human ear. As they penetrate through the skin down to deeper levels of the body, the sound waves give off heat when they reach a hard structure such as bone, and so this therapy is used to gently warm the surfaces of joints which might be inflamed, as in arthritis. Another method – diathermy – uses radio waves, the energy of which is converted into heat in deep tissues, leaving the skin cool. It is the same principle by which microwave cooking is done – from the inside out.

Ice treatment

Surprisingly, perhaps, cold is equally effective and can be tried if heat does not work in relieving pain – especially in muscles and joints. It is best to use a piece of ice without any sharp edges, somewhat in the shape of a large piece of soap. This can be made by putting water into a saucer or a small deep bowl and then freezing it. Remember to get rid of the sharp edges by letting them melt a little by running water on them. The ice should always be wrapped in a cloth because, like a hot-water bottle, it can burn the skin. Alternatively, you can use ice cubes in a rubber ice bag.

The ice, whether as a large, wrapped piece or in an ice bag, should be slowly and gently moved over the tender or painful part, this action being continued until you feel the skin go numb. It must not be done for more than five minutes at a time, and there should be at least a ten-minute rest in between, in case frostbite develops. Because of this danger, I do not advise this method being used in children, because of their relatively small size, unless proper medical advice has first been obtained.

You usually feel a number of sensations before the part goes numb. First, cold will be felt, then there may be a burning feeling, a stiffness in the tissues and finally numbness develops. Once this stage has been reached, the ice should be removed from the skin and you should move the affected part. The use of ice is particularly beneficial in obtaining movement in sore, stiff or painful limbs, hands and feet; and helps to lessen the pain of bruises, hangovers and headaches, in particular. It is not as useful on the larger parts of the body because of the much greater areas of flesh that have to be cooled.

It is thought that, in addition to its local anaesthetic qualities, the effects of ice are similar to those of acupuncture (pages 103–5) and TENS therapy (pages 100–2). This relationship was demonstrated in two studies published by Prof Ronald Melzack and others in 1980. In the first, patients suffering acute dental pain were given ice massage on the backs of their hands, on the same side as the pain, and surprisingly, the pain decreased in intensity by at least 50 per cent in the majority of the patients. In the other study, patients suffering from chronic low back pain were treated with both TENS therapy and ice massage, and it was found that both methods were equally effective and the ice treatment even more so in some patients.

Counter-irritants

There are a number of methods of relieving pain which depend on producing another type of injury to the skin, which acts as a counter-irritant to the original pain. The mustard plaster applied to the chest has been used for centuries for the pain of pleurisy (and is still occasionally used today). The old English method of dry needling for relieving painful rheumatic nodules, and the old methods which go under the name of 'cupping' are other outmoded examples of counter-irritants. In the latter, hot water is placed in a cup which is then emptied and its mouth quickly placed over the skin; as the cup cools, the air inside contracts, sucks the skin into the cup, damages it slightly, makes it painful and relieves the initial pain in the skin. Other traditional methods include poultices and fomentations (the application of warm cloths). The efficacy of such ancient Chinese practices as moxibustion (in which cones of the dried leaves of the herb *artemisia moxa* are burned almost down to the skin) and acupuncture (see pages 103–5) is wholly or partly based on their properties of counter-irritation.

Anything that has a counter-irritant effect on the skin stimulates the nerves in that area – thus acting in a similar way to TENS therapy (see pages 100–2) – and also expands the diameters of blood vessels and therefore increases the blood flow in the affected skin, which then becomes reddened and warm. It may be that a different sort of mild pain masks the initial pain, or that the pain-relieving effect is achieved because you feel that something positive has been done.

One of the most common counter-irritants available over the counter today is liniment – a medical preparation that is rubbed into the skin. It is generally used to sooth muscular aches and pain, but can also help arthritic joints. In addition to the warmth it gives to the skin, it is also usually applied by massage (see page 111) which is very comforting. The most common types of liniment are the white, methyl salicylate (oil of wintergreen), terebinthinae (turpentine) and saponis (soap) varieties. There are stronger ones which have a local anaesthetic effect and temporarily numb the nerve endings in the skin; these are sometimes used to relieve itching and some are so powerful that they can blister the skin. Liniment should never be used on broken skin, such as after the injury from a graze or a burn, or on sensitive areas, like the nipples. Those with sensitive skin or who get eczema should always consult their doctor before using it, and you should also check with your doctor before rubbing liniment on a strain or sprain to make sure that you will not be masking the pain of a fracture.

USEFUL ADDRESSES

I hope that in the preceding chapters I have answered most of your questions about pain and allayed some of your fears. I have already mentioned many of the most likely sources of help for your pain: you yourself, your family doctor, physiotherapists and other professional specialists. In this appendix are listed the names and addresses of organizations which should be able to help you further.

BRITAIN

Aleph One (biofeedback)
The Old Courthouse
High Street
Bottisham
Cambridge CB5 9BA

Arthritis and Rheumatism Council
  also at same address:
  British League against Rheumatism and
  British Association of Rheumatology and Rehabilitation
41 Eagle Street
London WC1R 4AR

Arthritis Care
6 Grosvenor Crescent
London SW1X 7ER

Back Pain Association
31–33 Park Road
Teddington
Middlesex TW11 8AB

British Heart Foundation
102 Gloucester Place
London W1H 4DH

British Medical Acupuncture Society
77–79 Chancery Lane
London WC2

British Migraine Association
178A High Road
Byfleet
Weybridge
Surrey KT14 7ED

British School of Osteopathy
1 Suffolk Street
London SW1

Cancer Aftercare and Rehabilitation Society
Lodge Cottage
Church Lane
Timsbury
Bath BA3 1LF

Chest Heart and Stroke Association
Tavistock House North
Tavistock Square
London WC1H 9JE

Horder Centre for Arthritics
St John's Road
Crowborough
East Sussex TN6 1XP

Migraine Trust
45 Great Ormond Street
London WC1N 3HD

National Childbirth Trust
9 Queensborough Terrace
Bayswater
London W2 3TB

National Society for Cancer Relief
Michael Sobell House
30 Dorset Square
London NW1 6QL

Relaxation for Living
29 Burwood Park Road
Walton-on-Thames
Surrey KT12 5LH

Women's National Cancer Control
 Campaign
1 South Audley Street
London W1X 5DG

UNITED STATES

Acupuncture International Association
2330 S Brentwood Boulevard
St Louis, MO 63144

American Guild of Hypnotherapists
7117 Farnam Street
Omaha, NE 68132

American Heart Association
7320 Greenville Avenue
Dallas, TX 75231

American Osteopathic Association
212 East Ohio Street
Chicago, IL 60611

American Pain Society
340 Kingsland Street
Nutley, NJ 07110

American Rheumatism Association
also **Arthritis Foundation**
3400 Peachtree Road, NE
Atlanta, GA 30326

American Society of Clinical
 Hypnosis
2250 E Devon Avenue, Suite 336
Des Plaines, IL 60018

Biofeedback Society of America
c/o Francine Butler, PhD

4301 Owens Street
Wheat Ridge, CO 80033

Childbirth without Pain Education
 Association
20134 Snowden
Detroit, MI 48235

International Association for the
 Study of Pain
Westlund Building, Room 301
1309 Summit Avenue
Seattle, WA 98101

National Committee on the
 Treatment of Intractable Pain
PO Box 9553
Friendship Station
Washington, DC 20016

National Migraine Foundation
5252 N Western Avenue
Chicago, IL 60625

CANADA

Acupuncture Foundation of Canada
10 St Mary Street
Toronto, ON
M4Y 1P9

Arthritis Society
1129 Carling Avenue
Ottawa, ON
K1Y 4G6

Arthritis Society
895 West Tenth Avenue
Vancouver, BC
V5Z 1L7

Arthritis Society
920 Yonge Street
Toronto, ON
M4W 3C7

Canadian Heart Foundation
1 Nicholas Street
Suite 1200

Ottawa, ON
K1N 7B7

Canadian Osteopathic Aid Society
575 Waterloo Street
London, ON
N6B 2R2

Canadian Physiotherapy Association
44 Eglinton Avenue West
Suite 201
Toronto, ON
M4R 1A1

Childbirth Education Association Toronto
33 Price Street
Suite 100
Toronto, ON
M4W 1Z2

L'Institut International du Stress
659 Hilton Street
Montreal, PQ
H2X 1W6

Migraine Foundation
390 Brunswick Street
Toronto, ON
M5R 2Z4

Ontario Osteopathic Society
45 Richmond Street West
Suite 401
Toronto, ON
M5H 1Z2

AUSTRALIA

Arthritis and Rheumatism Council
Wynyard House
291 George Street
Sydney
NSW 2000

Australian Arthritis and Rheumatism Foundation
The Queen Elizabeth Hospital
Woodville
South Australia 5011

Biofeedback Meditation Relaxation Centre
165 Adderton Road,
Carlingford
NSW 2118

Canberra Arthritis and Rheumatism Association
PO Box 352
Woden
ACT 2806

National Heart Foundation of Australia
55 Townshend Street
Phillip
ACT 2606

NEW ZEALAND

Arthritis and Rheumatism Foundation of New Zealand
PO Box 10–020
Southern Cross Building
Brandon Street
Wellington

National Heart Foundation of New Zealand
17 Great South Road
Newmarket
PO Box 17128
Green Lane
Auckland 5

SOUTH AFRICA

National Heart Effort
PO Box 70
Tygerberg

South Africa Rheumatism and Arthritis Association
Namaqua House
36 Burg Street
Capetown 8001

INTERNATIONAL DRUG-NAME EQUIVALENTS

Generic name	UK trade name	Australia trade name	US trade name	Canada trade name
acyclovir	Zovirax		Zovirax	Zovirax
buprenorphine hydrochloride	Temgesic	Temgesic		
carbamazepine	Tegretol	Convuline Tegretol	Tegretol	Tegretol Apo–Carbamazepine Mazepine
clonidine hydrochloride	Catapres Dixarit	Catapres Dixarit	Catapres	Catapres Dixarit
codeine phosphate	generic only	Codlin	generic only	Paveral
cortisone acetate	Cortisyl Cortistab Cortelan	Cortone Cortate	Cortistan Cortone Acetate Pantisone Adricort	Cortone
benorylate benorilate (US)	}Benoral Triadol	Benoral		
dextropropoxyphene propoxyphene (US, Canada)	Doloxene (as napsylate)	Doloxene (as napsylate)	Ropoxy Dolene Plain Darvon Harmar SK-65 Profene 65 Paragesic 65 (all as hydrochloride) Darvon-N (as napsylate)	Novopropoxyn 642 (both as hydrochloride) Darvon-N (as napsylate)
ergotamine tartrate	Lingraine Medihaler-Ergotamine	Lingraine	Ergomar Ergostat Medihaler-Ergotamine Wigrettes	Ergomar Gynergen Medihaler-Ergotamine
ergotamine-containing suppositories	Cafergot	Cafergot-PB		Cafergot Cafergot-PB

Generic name	UK trade name	Australia trade name	US trade name	Canada trade name
fenoprofen calcium	Fenopron Fenopron D Progesic	Fenopron	Nalfon	Nalfon
halothane	Fluothane	Fluothane	Fluothane	Fluothane Somnothane
hydrocortisone sodium succinate	Solu-Cortef Corlan Efcortelan Soluble	Solu-Cortef Efcortelan Soluble Nordicort	A-Hydrocort Solu-Cortef Hycorace	Solu-Cortef S-Cortilean
ibuprofen	Apsifen Brufen Ebufac Ibu-Slo Maxagesic Nurofen Proflex Uniprofen	Brufen Inflam	Motrin Rufen	Amersol Motrin
idoxuridine	Dendrid Herpid Idoxene Iduridin Kerecid Ophthalmadine	Herplex Herplex-D Stoxil	Dendrid Herplex Stoxil	Herplex Herplex-D Stoxil
indomethacin	Artracin Imbrilon Indocid Indocid-R Indoflex Indolar Indolar SR Mobilan	Indocid Rheumacin	Indocin Indocin SR	Indocid Indocid SR Novomethacin
pentazocine	Fortral (as lactate & hydrochloride)	Fortral (as lactate & hydrochloride)	Talwin (as lactate & hydrochloride)	Talwin (as lactate & hydrochloride)
pizotifen pizotyline (US, Canada)	Sandomigran	Sandomigran		Sandomigran Sandomigran DS
promazine hydrochloride	Sparine	Sparine	Sparine Norazine Prozine	Sparine

ACKNOWLEDGEMENTS

I am indebted to Prof Ronald Melzack both for writing a foreword to the US and Canadian editions, and for his kind permission to reproduce a section of the McGill–Melzack Pain Questionnaire on page 18, as well as to use his research information for the diagrams on pages 19, 25 (top), 37, 75 and 81.

I am very grateful to Prof Tess O'Rourke Brophy for her foreword to the Australian edition.

I would also like to acknowledge the valuable support of my friend and colleague Dr Christopher Wells, present Director of the Centre of Pain Relief, Walton Hospital, Liverpool.

Finally, my thanks are due to my editors, Piers Murray Hill and Nancy Duin, and to my publisher, Martin Dunitz, for their help and encouragement.

Sampson Lipton, 1984

The publishers would like to thank the following individuals and organizations for their permission to reproduce photographs: Julie Habel/Art Directors Photo Library, London (page 41); Department of Medical Photography, Colchester District, and the British Medical Acupuncture Society (page 103); Pictor International, London (pages 84 and 99). The cover photo is courtesy Heinz Schwarz/Pictor International, London.

The studio photographs were taken by Dave Brown. The modelling was done by Roy Seeley and Joanna Parker, under the expert supervision of physiotherapists Helen Shilston and Bridget Ellis of Westminster Hospital. The props were kindly supplied by the following organizations: Bed linen by Dorma, Manchester; the footstool and rocking chair by Harrods, London; the bed by the London Bedding Centre, London SW1; the china and glass by the Reject Shop, Kings Road, London.

The diagrams were drawn by Cathy Clench and Terry Carriage.

INDEX

Page numbers in *italic* refer to the illustrations.

30; shingles, 90; simple painkillers, 92–3
dysmenorrhoea, 9, 79–80

elbow joint, 26
electrical stimulation therapy, 100–2, 104, 111, 112; *102*
epesiotomy, 83
epidural anaesthesia, 82–4, 90, 98
ergotamine tartrate, 67–8, 69
exercise, 108–11; back pain, 54–5; *52*; heart disease, 61; osteoarthritis, 27–8; rheumatic disease, 30–1; *32–5*
eyesight, and headaches, 72

facial nerve pain, 85
fenoprofen, 30
fibrositis, 29
fingers: exercises, 31; *34*; joints, 24; *25*
food: headaches, 71; migraine, 65; *66*

gallstones, 86–7; *87*
gastritis, 86
gastroenteritis, 86
gate control, 10, 100, 104, 111
gold injections, 30
gout, 29; *29*
gumboils, 76, 77

hands, exercises, 31; *34*
hangovers, 71
head: anatomy, 36–7; exercises, 31; *32*; nerve pain, 51; rheumatic nodules, 51
headache, 6, 7, 21, 64–72
heart attacks, 57, 59–60, 92; *60*
heart disease, 9, 57–61, 103
heartburn, 86
heat treatment, 111–12; *110*
herpes simplex, 78
herpes zoster, 89–90
hiatus hernia, 85–6
high blood pressure, *72*
hip joints, 24–6, 30
'housemaid's knee', 30
hydrotherapy, 55
hypnosis, 20, 105, 106
hypnotics, 94–5

ibuprofen, 79
ice treatment, 112
indomethacin, 30, 54, 79
inflammation, 9; back pain, 42–3; drug treatment, 30; rheumatoid arthritis, 28

joints, 24–6; *25*; exercise, 106–7; gout, 29; locked, 43; osteoarthritis, 26–8; rheumatoid arthritis, 28; surgical replacement, 30

kinins, 9, 111
knee joints, 26; *25*

labour pains, *see* childbirth
laminectomy, 48
legs: atherosclerosis, 61–2; *63*; exercises, 31; *35*
Librium, 20
ligaments, torn, 43
liniment, 113
locked joints, 43
lumbago, 39
lumbar spondylosis, 48–9, 50; *49*

McGill Pain Questionnaire, 16–17, 73, 81; *18–19, 25, 37, 75, 81*
manipulation, 54
MAOIs, 96–7
massage, 54, 111; *110*
measurement of pain, 16–19; *17, 18–19*
mefenamic acid, 79
menopause, 26–7
meptazinol, 93
methysergide, 68, 69
metoclopramide, 67
migraine, 64–8, 104, 106; *66*
modulation, 15–16
mood and pain, 19–21
morphine, 20, 93–4
mouth ulcers, 78
muscles, 26; exercise, 55, 106–7; rheumatic nodules, 51–3; rheumatism, 24, 29; tears, 43

naproxen, 30
narcotics, 93–4

121

women: childbirth, 19, 80–4, 101, 104; *81*; migraine, 64, 66; osteoarthritis, 26–7; period pain, 9, 79–80, 102; Raynaud's disease, 62; rheumatic arthritis, 28

X-rays, disc disease, 47–8

yoga, 106, 109

Other books in the Positive Health Guide Series

MIGRAINE & HEADACHES
Understanding, controlling and avoiding the pain
Dr Marcia Wilkinson

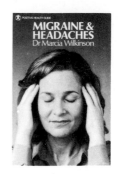

An eminent migraine clinic director explains what makes migraine different from other headaches, how you can identify and avoid the causes of your attacks, and what you can do to deal with the pain. Featuring special easy-to-follow relaxation exercises this is an indispensable book for every migraine and headache sufferer.

OVERCOMING ARTHRITIS
A guide to coping with stiff or aching joints
Dr Frank Dudley Hart

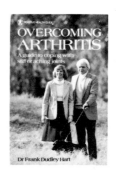

A world-renowned rheumatologist brings fresh hope for the millions who suffer from arthritis and rheumatism. Dozens of practical hints and gadgets are illustrated for coping with arthritis in everyday life and around the home. Special exercises are demonstrated to ease stiffening joints.

THE BACK – RELIEF FROM PAIN
Patterns of back pain – how to deal with and avoid them
Dr Alan Stoddard

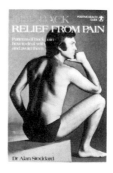

A leading osteopathic physician shows how to overcome back pain, and even more important, how to look after your back to see that it does not let you down. Packed with practical hints and simple exercises that can be done at home.

The British School of Osteopathy

* 2 9 4 6 *

This book is to be returned on or before
the last date stamped below.

1 1 JAN 1988

1 8 JAN 1988

18 DEC 1989
-2 DEC 1994
1 4 FEB 2012
2 0 JUN 2018

LIPTON, S.